Praise for Joey Miller

"I have worked with Joey Miller as both an obstetrician working in Chicago and as a patient myself. It was because of Joey that I was able to return to delivering babies in the very hospital I lost my own. I know [this book] will help women who are grieving as well as the health professionals who grieve alongside them but often struggle with how best to support their patients emotionally."

—Gwyneth Bryant, MD, Obstetrician/Gynecologist, Prentice Women's Hospital, Chicago, and Clinical Instructor of Obstetrics and Gynecology, Northwestern Feinberg School of Medicine, Chicago

"I have worked with Joey Miller for over a decade, and in that time, I have seen the benefits that women and their partners accrue by being in her care. [This book will] make a valuable contribution to the many individuals (patients, families, care providers) who may never have the chance to work with her on a personal basis."

—William Grobman, MD, MBA, Northwestern Memorial Hospital, and Professor of Obstetrics and Gynecology and Preventative Medicine, Northwestern Feinberg School of Medicine, Chicago

"Joey Miller is Chicago's 'go-to' source for perinatal loss counseling. Ms. Miller has tremendous depth of experience with patients whose grief originates within a variety of different contexts. My endorsement reflects the clinical experience of years of patients who have benefitted from her care in the most trying of circumstances. I trust her advice, respect her insight, and am glad that she wishes to share her knowledge with a broader audience."

—Cassing Hammond, MD, Director, Section and Fellowship in Family Planning, Associate Professor of Obstetrics and Gynecology, Northwestern Feinberg School of Medicine, Chicago

"Joey Miller is an exceptional clinician and therapist. She has expert diagnostic acumen accompanied by unparalleled compassion and fortitude that allow her to walk with her patients in times of profound loss, horrific tragedy, and immeasurable threats to themselves and those they love. Her capacity to hold patients in a loving and safe space while also holding them accountable to their own aspirations and goals is inspiring. I am profoundly grateful to be able to learn from her and work with her in the care of individuals who are suffering."

—Elizabeth Kieff, MD, Psychiatrist, Private Practice, formerly Student Affairs Dean, Faculty Member, and University Student Mental Health Psychiatrist, Department of Psychiatry, The University of Chicago, Chicago

"Joey Miller is a locally and nationally recognized expert and respected advocate, therapeutic practitioner, and incredibly regarded presenter in the area of perinatal loss. Much of her professional career also includes educating as well as supporting the physicians, nurses, and support staff that care for these patients and families."

—Susan Rizzato, MSW, LCSW, Perinatal Loss Program Coordinator, Northwestern Memorial Hospital, Chicago

"Joey Miller is a very competent and highly skilled clinician who joins her clients and their stories of loss, suffering, and adversity in empathic and compassionate ways. She connects with clients while building resiliency and hope for their futures. Joey is highly regarded among colleagues and clients and their families who continue to seek her out not only during vulnerable times in their lives but also in their journey of remembering, meaning making, and resiliency."

—Denada Hoxha, PhD, Psychologist, Private Practice, and Professor, Loyola University, Chicago

"Joey Miller is brilliant in her vocation and seeks to bring healing and peace to all who seek her comfort and guidance. This tremendous book flows from years of experience—action put into words. Joey Miller is an angel of hope in the midst of the pain and tragedies of life."

—Very Rev. Gregory Sakowicz, Rector, Holy Name Cathedral Parish, Chicago

Rebirth

JOEY MILLER, MSW, LCSW

Rebirth

THE JOURNEY OF PREGNANCY
AFTER A LOSS

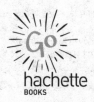

hachette
BOOKS

New York

Copyright © 2020 by Joey Miller

Cover design by Terri Sirma
Cover illustration © Nechayka/Shutterstock
Cover copyright © 2020 by Hachette Book Group, Inc.

Hachette Go, an imprint of Hachette Books
Hachette Book Group
1290 Avenue of the Americas
New York, NY 10104
HachetteGo.com
Facebook.com/HachetteGo
Instagram.com/HachetteGo

First Edition: October 2020

Hachette Books is a division of Hachette Book Group, Inc.

The Hachette Go and Hachette Books name and logos are trademarks of Hachette Book Group, Inc.

The publisher is not responsible for websites (or their content) that are not owned by the publisher.

Print book interior design by Amy Quinn

Library of Congress Cataloging-in-Publication Data
Names: Miller, Joey, author.
Title: Rebirth : the journey of pregnancy after a loss / Joey Miller, MSW, LCSW.
Description: First edition. | New York: Hachette Go, [2020] | Includes bibliographical references and index. |
Identifiers: LCCN 2020025920 | ISBN 9780306846618 (trade paperback) | ISBN 9780306846625 (ebook)
Subjects: LCSH: Pregnancy. | Pregnancy--Complications.
Classification: LCC RG551 .M55 2020 | DDC 618.2--dc23
LC record available at https://lccn.loc.gov/2020025920

ISBNs: 978-0-306-84661-8 (paperback); 978-0-306-84662-5 (ebook)

Printed in the United States of America

LSC-C

10 9 8 7 6 5 4 3 2 1

Contents

Author's Note

THE USE OF THE WORD *physician* throughout this book is intended to imply any primary medical provider, whether that person is a medical doctor, an advanced practice nurse (nurse practitioner, certified nurse midwife), etc. Also, the narratives in this book are real and reflect twenty-five different women's experiences with loss and subsequent pregnancy. The majority of women chose to use their given first names; a minority have been respectfully changed to maintain anonymity per individual request.

Foreword

As AN OBSTETRICIAN, I HAVE the best job in the world. Witnessing the miracle of birth is something I have learned to never take for granted as pregnancy does not always work out the way it is supposed to. It is a hard and awful truth that pregnancies can develop complications, end prematurely, and in some cases babies die. And it is far more common than people perceive: a loss can occur with or without warning and at any time during all three trimesters, at delivery, or postpartum. According to the Mayo Clinic, an estimated 10 to 20 percent of pregnancies prior to twenty weeks end in loss. The Centers for Disease Control and Prevention indicates that stillbirth after twenty weeks' gestation affects 1 in 100 pregnancies. Some are associated with birth defects or chromosomal abnormalities, such as Down syndrome, and others occur in patients with high-risk conditions, such as diabetes or hypertension; but 25 percent or more of stillbirths occur without any explanation. No matter how or when their loss occurred, all parents want to know why this happened, and it is very frustrating to tell them that medical knowledge currently cannot always answer this question. Hopefully, one day we will understand more about why some pregnancies end before full gestation and why some babies die after delivery.

I have been practicing high-risk obstetrics for over thirty years now, and with that territory comes the inevitability of caring for patients whose baby has died. The skill of breaking bad news and comforting patients was not taught in medical school, so many of us physicians have to develop it by intuition, trial and error, and watching others. Over the years, my patients have taught me most of what I now know. I have learned that most women have overwhelming guilt, which tortures them for a long time, with such recurring thoughts as "if only I had not worked so much, if only we had not had sex the night before, if only I had not fallen asleep on my back," and so on. I also have learned that the most important thing for all women to hear is, "This was not your fault." Losing a child is not fair, and there is never a good reason for it to happen. Making sure we convey this to women who are grieving is one of the most important parts of care. Another important part of care is discussing future pregnancies with women who have undergone a loss. It can be a difficult subject, but necessary.

Fortunately, there are counselors who are experienced in perinatal loss. These counselors provide crisis intervention, supportive counseling, and education to women who experience pregnancy and infant loss. They can also play a role in educating nurses and physicians how they may best support these patients in the aftermath of their loss. I have the highest respect for these perinatal grief counselors, who perform this difficult but incredibly valuable task day after day. Joey Miller is one of those extraordinary individuals, but her experience far exceeds years in the hospital or clinic settings where, for many women, the grief is only just beginning. A mental health professional, Joey has extensive experience supporting bereaved women and families in the weeks, months, sometimes years following their loss and as women battle trauma, depression, and anxiety. And she has provided expert guidance when those women are ready to consider the unthinkable—conceiving again. Joey is much respected for her expertise in this area; many practitioners refer their patients to her knowing that they will receive the best care and comfort possible. I have witnessed the difference Joey makes in the lives of people who are going through this difficult time, and how they come back stronger.

Joey understands the devastating nature of perinatal loss as well as its long-lasting effects. She has helped families learn to cope with the fear that comes with contemplating another pregnancy, the sadness on anniversaries of the loss, and the anxiety and panic that ensue as the patient not only approaches the point in the next pregnancy where the prior one was lost, but also until that woman gets well beyond delivery.

Joey has also been part of the joy as well as the mixed emotions that can emerge after a subsequent successful pregnancy. She assists and helps manage the realities of parenting a child after identity and confidence have been so compromised by prior loss. Joey shares all of this knowledge in this book, ensuring no woman has to go through any of this alone, and easing the journey through this dark place. By sharing her experiences and those of her patients, she extends a hand to those in need. This book is not only for women who have experienced a pregnancy or infant loss and who are conceiving again; physicians and nurses will benefit as well from reading it. Whether you are a patient or provider, my hope for you is that reading this book will bring some measure of comfort, strength, and emotional support and guidance.

Alan Peaceman, MD,
Professor and Chief, Division of Maternal Fetal Medicine,
Department of Obstetrics and Gynecology,
Northwestern Feinberg School of Medicine
Chicago, Illinois

Introduction

My Hope for You

THE VIEW FROM MY OFFICE window is far and wide across the landscape. From where I sit, I see the road on which many travel, off into the warm and golden sunlight, cradling a new and healthy life in their arms. I also see the vast expanse of space that runs from this road all the way up to my office door. Much of that land is a graveyard, filled with remembrances of a lost pregnancy or baby, and now, the painful memories of all the hopes and dreams that were connected to that child's life and future. The mothers and fathers of those babies will not continue on that road as expected, planned, or as desired; the path they believed and trusted would lead to parenthood. Instead, they have been thrown mercilessly from that road and abruptly learn there will be no continuing pregnancy, no baby, and no future with that child. This reality is the shocking and harsh aftermath of perinatal loss—the death of a baby during pregnancy, labor and delivery, the postpartum period, or early infancy.

For nearly twenty years, I have and continue to receive thousands of parents at my door who are gravely wounded and devastated, sometimes even feeling dead themselves after having just lost their baby. I have compassionately welcomed and worked tirelessly with them, for days, for months, and even years, to treat and care for their unbelievably complex injuries from this loss but to also help them gradually and eventually find their way back to that road.

The mere thought of starting that journey again can seem an absolute impossibility—unsafe and threatening, and filled with dread. However, from all that I have seen, I know that it is not. It is very, very difficult, but it is not impossible. The parents I meet are consumed by profound tragedy, as well as aching from the gaping wounds created by heartbreak. In my world, and from all I have seen firsthand, there is nothing, *nothing*, worse than losing a baby or child. Because the extent of the injuries is tremendous, my patients initially (but understandably) cannot see anything beyond the loss of their pregnancy and the death of their baby.

If you are one of those innocent and tragic victims, you already know there is absolutely nothing, *not one single thing* I can say that will lessen the pain of what you are experiencing. The *only* thing that would genuinely help is for you to still be pregnant and still have your baby. I am profoundly sorry for the reason our paths have crossed, and while I am glad you have picked up this book, I wish our connection had occurred under very different circumstances. I know you face an uncertain road ahead, but you do not have to walk it alone.

Although it may be impossible to imagine that you will ever find your way through your intense and immense grief, much less back to that road toward parenthood, I know from experience that eventually you can and will. The reason I know this is possible is that I see parents go on to find happiness and joy in their lives again, although never forgetting about their lost pregnancy or their deceased baby. I see them become empowered and find ways to return to that road, continue, *and then complete* their journey to parenthood and family growth. I know because this is my professional life's work. I consider it a privilege to partner with women and their families on this journey, and am always touched when contacted with news of the healthy delivery of a subsequent baby. We joyously celebrate that new life, and we also remember and cherish the baby (or babies) who came before.

Over the years, I have learned so much more than I have taught, and I have my patients to thank for that. I have learned all the things that were not helpful for parents, and many of the things that were. I learned how to sit and listen to the aching and raw emotion of the loss. I learned how to help parents sort it, process it, and understand it. I learned how to care for wounds before scar tissue begins to form. I learned how to teach parents to find ways to carry their deceased baby in their hearts, honoring and remembering him or her. I learned how to help parents confront their worst fears and work through them and then beyond them.

As inconceivable as it seems, I also learned how to help them find their way back to that terrifying and uncertain road, identify another entry point, and resume their journey. I learned how to help parents pace themselves through the days and weeks and months and years ahead, advising them of the inevitable sharp curves before them so they will not be blindsided or feel as unprepared again. Over the years, I learned more and more, and eventually, I found a way to help turn thousands of parents' grief into something beautiful and meaningful. I used all that I learned to create a road map so that people like you wouldn't have to feel so lost, so afraid, and so very alone. It is my hope and intention that this book will guide and support you through that process.

Through the years, I have counseled thousands of incredibly brave women who first came to my office, seeking solace after a tragedy. Twenty-five of these women—women who lost a pregnancy or baby and went on to confront their deepest fears by considering and then embarking on a subsequent pregnancy—have graciously agreed to publicly share parts of their experiences to raise awareness, educate others, provide support and guidance, and most important, to encourage hope. Each woman's path is highly individual and reflects the intensely personal nature of grief, depression, anxiety, fear, and trauma. Many have decided to use their real first names; a number have chosen to remain anonymous. Their narratives, interlaced between the concrete guidance presented, recount how their lives are changed forever by loss, *and* they also provide striking evidence that there *is* life beyond loss. Their words capture moments of desperation and hopelessness, the agony of uncertainty, and the growing pains critical to their own rebirth.

The book you hold, *Rebirth*, reveals *how* these women found—and now how *you* can find—your way back to that road: from the point of unimaginable grief and tragedy, to better understanding and processing of your emotions, to exploring time-sensitive choices ahead of you as you consider the daunting and overwhelming task of trying again. Further, this book will guide you through every step of your next pregnancy, and help empower you to eventually embrace that new and growing life, as well as your life *and yourself* after the loss.

No matter where you're currently at in your journey—whether your loss just occurred, or whether you're subsequently pregnant—you, your partner, and your medical providers can all benefit from this book. The chapters will guide you every step of the way through the process from the decision to try again and what may unfold for you emotionally as you move through three trimesters, delivery, and then eventually postpartum. By starting at the beginning, you will gain a deeper perspective of the challenges you've already faced or are currently facing, which will inevitably help with those ahead. The insight offered will undoubtedly improve your sightlines—and thus confidence—as you continue to make decisions long into your future.

Still, it's normal to have doubts; you will continue to have many fears; for a time, you may have lost hope—that's all to be expected given what you have been through. Walking by faith is considerably more difficult than walking by sight. What matters now is that you're no longer alone in the dark, without anyone who speaks the same language as you in the place of raw grief. Please know I have a light and I know the way well. I will walk as slowly and cautiously as you need, but I will also walk confidently. And, we can walk together.

Facing the Aftermath of Tragedy

Totally Unprepared

In your chest of drawers,
Your clothes were clean
Your diapers awaiting use
Your blankets were warm and ready
Your dad put on the finishing touches
assembling the bassinet and stroller,
safety seat in the car.

Your toys were ready to be played with
Your books were waiting to be read
The rocking chair stood idle as it waited
We waited with great anticipation.
We were prepared.

Yet we could not know what that day would hold
the shock
the horror of silence
We could not prepare

our hearts
to be shattered
We were caught totally unprepared.

Totally unprepared for the pain of losing you
Totally unprepared for the travail of delivering you
Totally unprepared for the look of loss in your father's eyes
in my eyes
in the eyes of grandma and grandpa and nana.

Totally unprepared to let you go.

　　　　—**BRITTANY**

PREGNANCY IS SUPPOSED TO BE a happy, exciting, and joyful experience. Even the actual words used to express the news—*"I'm expecting"*—denote that a healthy, full-term delivery is anticipated. Unfortunately, even if you were able to conceive spontaneously and straightforwardly, the happily-ever-after is abruptly and dramatically interrupted when the miracle of pregnancy is transformed into the nightmare of loss. You're left facing not only the physical loss of this much-desired pregnancy and baby, but also the loss of the expected future, as well as loss of control, loss of time, loss of clarity, loss of confidence, and loss of identity. *You were expecting to be a mother.* The complete story is not supposed to end this way.

Sadly, babies can and sometimes do die during all three trimesters of pregnancy, during labor and delivery, the postpartum period, and early infancy. In 2010 (most current data available), there were an estimated 6.2 million pregnancies conceived in the United States. Of this total, 4 million had a live birth outcome.[1] In the United States in 2018, there were 3.8 million live births reported, a number relatively unchanged.[2] These statistics suggest that approximately 2.2 million pregnancies annually end in loss in the United States. For further reference, in the United States:

- An estimated 10 to 20% of known pregnancies end in miscarriage (loss prior to 20 weeks' gestation). That risk increases with age. At age 40, the risk is about 40%; at age 45, it is 80%. And, approximately 50% of miscarriages are associated with a chromosomal abnormality.[3]

- 1 in 100 pregnancies end in stillbirth (loss after 20 weeks' gestation); this is about 24,000 deaths annually.[4]
- There are an additional 22,000 infant deaths a year (death of a child less than 1 year of age).[5]
- 1 in 10 babies is born preterm (prior to 37 weeks' gestation).[6]
- Congenital malformations, preterm birth and low birth weight, maternal pregnancy complications, and sudden infant death syndrome (SIDS) are the leading causes of infant mortality in the United States.[7]

The numbers further explode when viewed internationally:
- According to the World Health Organization (WHO), there are over 6.3 million perinatal deaths a year worldwide. Of these, 2.64 million are stillbirths, and 3.0 million are early neonatal deaths (loss occurring within the first month of life).[8]
- In 2017, the WHO reported there were 4.1 million infant deaths worldwide (death of a child less than 1 year of age).[9]

Although many advances have been made to enhance and improve perinatal care, these losses can occur with or without warning, and with a staggering frequency. They can occur due to complications of placenta, cord, or membranes; infection and injury; chromosomal and congenital anomalies (that have a genetic, environmental, or unknown cause); or due to other maternal health issues. Independent of how or when they occur, they *all* represent an extraordinary disruption in the path a pregnant woman was expecting to pursue for herself, her family, and her life. When that happens, she, and in this case *you*, are caught totally unprepared.

EMOTIONAL FREE FALL

Everyone who has lost a pregnancy or baby quickly learns you don't hit rock bottom immediately. The shock of loss can feel devastating, but initially, there are distractions, and decisions to be made (for example, *"What happens next?"*

"Will I need medication, a surgical procedure, or to go through delivery?" "What will happen to the baby's body?"). The shock is accompanied by feelings of profound disappointment, sadness, loneliness, anger, jealousy, helplessness, and hopelessness.

You may also struggle with anxiety, finding it challenging to manage feelings of worry, fear, uncertainty, an admitted lack of control, and an unknown future. You may wonder whether you will ever be able to see through this unimaginable weight of grief. Your frame of reference is now loss. It doesn't matter that the majority of women have healthy pregnancies and deliveries; you did not.

The emerging reality is, you have been cheated out of a healthy, happy pregnancy, an exciting and joyful delivery, and the experience of raising this baby in early infancy. You have learned firsthand that cruel and ironic twists of fate can occur. Optimistic expectations can be shattered, and bad outcomes are a real possibility, not only something that happens to someone else. Then, it gets worse.

Confusion and chaos begin to set in. You grow dizzy and disoriented, trying hard to make sense of something that doesn't make any sense at all. The world you once knew, believed in, and counted on has changed dramatically. This is where the questions begin, and they often do not stop.

"Why (and how) did this happen?"
"Why now?"
"Why me, why us?"
"Why this pregnancy, this baby?"
"What did I do wrong?"
"Why wasn't this prevented?"
"How could I not have known?"
"Why couldn't I protect him/her?"

This is also where the feelings of guilt begin. Some women are eventually provided with answers as to the probable cause of their loss, but many more are left with unanswered questions they are forced to carry the rest of their lives. In the absence of a clear etiology, women often begin to question and then blame themselves. The reality is that you didn't do *anything* to cause your loss. There is *nothing* you did, didn't do, or could have done differently to prevent it. As you will continue to learn, the loss of pregnancy and the death of a baby are not discretionary; it can happen to anyone. *It just happened to you.* You who were prepared and waiting, wanting, and very willing to bring a baby into this world. It's a hard and harsh landing when you are forced to reenter that world, no longer pregnant, and without your baby. *This* is when you might truly hit rock bottom—in the days and weeks and months following your loss, and as the wake of tragedy widens.

ALL LOSSES ARE REAL

If you experienced an early loss such as a first trimester miscarriage, you may not feel justified in—and guilty about—your grief reactions, especially if others around you disenfranchise your feelings and experience on any level. You may also find yourself even more depressed, anxious, and angry because you are not able to express your feelings and have them legitimatized by others. Please know your loss is real—regardless of when or how it occurred—and it can affect your identity, confidence, and sense of control in the world.

If you experienced a tragic prenatal diagnosis and were in the heartbreaking position of having to choose between continuing your pregnancy or terminating, and you decided on the latter, your guilt may also be heavy. While you were forced to make a choice, on some level—and through circumstances entirely outside your control—you didn't feel as if you had much of a "choice" at all. You didn't choose to be in crisis or to face a prenatal diagnosis or condition that affected your pregnancy and baby. For many women, the "choice" was a decision between horrible and terrible. Although the end result was a premature end to your pregnancy, you likely focused on avoiding suffering, pain, or a compromised quality of life for your child. Given the circumstances, you made the best decision you could at the time with the information you had.

In both cases, these losses are real. You have every right to grieve the loss of this pregnancy, this baby, and the loss of the future you had planned with this child.

MARNEY

Our loss of our daughter occurred the night/early morning before our scheduled C-section. I couldn't sleep and went out to the couch to lie down. I remember feeling her kick and never thinking anything was wrong. I was so nervous about the surgery and making sure that my son was taken care of before we left, that I never realized I didn't feel her move that morning. When the nurse could not find her heartbeat on the monitor, I guided her to where I knew she was. It never even crossed my mind that anything was wrong ... we were in such shock. There was absolute silence: in our room, in our hearts, in our hopes for the future. We had no idea what had hit us ...

DEPRESSION, PTSD, AND LOSS

Depressive feelings are common and expected following the loss of a pregnancy or the death of a baby. However, the signs and symptoms of grief can look identical to those of clinical depression. According to the American Psychiatric Association,[10] criteria for clinical depression include at least five of the following symptoms that are experienced every day or nearly every day for a period of two weeks:

- Depressed mood
- Markedly diminished interest or pleasure in all or almost all activities
- Significant weight change (loss or gain) or appetite disturbance
- Insomnia or hypersomnia
- Psychomotor agitation or retardation
- Fatigue or loss of energy
- Feelings of worthlessness, or excessive or inappropriate guilt
- Diminished ability to think or concentrate; indecisiveness
- Recurrent thoughts of death, suicidal ideation

It's easy to see how a bereaved individual might experience these same symptoms. Initially, it is impossible to tease out whether your symptoms are based in grief, or reflective of clinical depression. Consulting with an experienced mental health provider who is well versed in grief/loss can help identify (and then treat) more severe reactions and provide support through the continued grief process. That person can also facilitate a referral to explore the possibility of medication for additional support if indicated.

FINDING AND CONFIRMING CONNECTION WITH A THERAPIST

There are times when it's not just useful, but imperative, to seriously consider individual therapy to help weather the emotional challenges you face. But finding a good therapist can feel overwhelming, especially if you don't know where or how to start. Here are ways to begin your search:

- Ask a trusted professional (OB/GYN, advanced practice nurse, internist, etc.) for referrals. Most maintain current lists or have trusted colleagues to whom they refer patients.
- Contact your closest major medical center's social work, psychology, or psychiatry department and ask for local referrals.
- Consider asking a friend or family member for a referral if they've had a personal (and positive) experience with a particular therapist or practice. Note: Some therapists will not treat members of the same family or may not believe themselves to be the best match for your situation. However, all can suggest alternative referrals if/as needed.
- Complete an online search through your insurance carrier or a reputable search engine, such as psychologytoday.com or psychology.com. Although online searches can be of use to many, there are two potential downsides to this approach. First, online searches for general providers (for example, within a specific zip code) can return an inordinate list of names, leaving you in the same position as when you first started. In this case, just pick several and place calls. See who gets back to you fastest and has availability that works with your schedule. Second, searching under specialty may be frustrating as many sites restrict the search field to a single prefixed category, such as "grief/loss," or "women's issues." Recognize these can be

(continues)

(continued)

broad categories within themselves, and the first person you contact who is experienced in grief/loss may not be in *pregnancy and infant loss*. Don't, however, immediately rule someone out if they don't have expertise in this exact area. While having previous clinical experience in loss and trauma is ideal, it's not essential. Many licensed quality providers may still be a good fit for you and can help. Begin making calls now.

Once you have secured your first appointment, think about how you ideally wish it to begin. Is it helpful for you to write down some points you want to cover and share those with the therapist at the start of the appointment? Or does that feel like too much pressure? It might be more helpful to begin that appointment with something like, *"I'm not at all sure where to start, and I'm feeling pretty disorganized. Will you please guide me with short questions and I can try to answer them?"*

Generally, first appointments cover introductions and begin obtaining some background history and information about where you're at right now. An hour can go by fast, and there's the potential to leave not knowing much about the therapist's personality and style, or how you feel about her or him. At the start of the first appointment, ask the therapist to reserve the last ten or fifteen minutes to obtain his or her feedback, which may include initial goals and a treatment plan. This can also help you confirm the therapist's understanding and perspective of where you're at and what you are willing to work on.

Pay attention to personality. Having a rapport and comfort level with this person early on is essential to the progress of your work. If you don't feel a connection within the first several appointments, say so. In so doing, you create an opportunity for both of you to discuss what might be going on. Sometimes this reaction is more a reflection of painful or uncomfortable session content than about the therapist. In this case, the therapist can make recommendations to make the work feel more manageable and tolerable, perhaps limiting the time spent on a particular topic during each session. And, in the event there really isn't a connection, the therapist may be able to identify alternative referrals for you, now armed with more clinical information about your circumstances.

That might feel disappointing to begin again, but it's worth the time invested in finding the right person for you.

Lastly, don't be discouraged if some therapists don't accept your insurance, have a long wait list, or are not accepting new patients. If you can schedule an appointment, do so, but in the interim, continue your search. You'll eventually find someone licensed and credentialed who will give you the support and guidance you need and deserve.

Along with the experience of profound tragedy, there can also exist the additional layer of trauma. Although historically diagnosed in veterans of the military, post-traumatic stress disorder (PTSD) is a condition that is becoming increasingly recognized and considered in the context of perinatal loss, as is acute stress disorder (ASD), a similar condition but with less intensity and duration than PTSD. Not every woman who experiences a perinatal loss will develop signs and symptoms of PTSD or ASD, but some do, and either of these disorders add another layer of challenge to a bereaved mother's existing grief. (I talk more about PTSD and ASD in Chapter 6.)

NAVIGATING ROCK BOTTOM

You are not the same person you were before your loss, even though you may physically look the same to others. There is no visible or obvious sign of your injuries as there would be had you fractured your femur and had your leg in a full cast. As you work to reenter your world, still with real injuries that are invisible to others, it can be difficult to know what to do and say to best care for and protect yourself during this time of increased vulnerability. You'll be doing this all while others are looking to you for guidance and support through their own grief reactions to your loss. You play the lead role here. Others will be wanting and expecting your continued presence in their lives as usual. That can feel—and is—overwhelming as you simultaneously work to find your footing in the early days, weeks, and months ahead. Although nothing and no one can prepare you to navigate some of the sharp curves ahead, knowledge of what's coming can be helpful.

Decisions Will Need to Be Made About Your Baby's Belongings

Most women, even in spite of religious traditions or personal superstitions, end up having some baby items at home before the actual delivery, and if you delivered, there are many still at home following your loss. Ask yourself what would feel worse: having these items around and staring you in the face, or having all traces of the baby removed? Both answers are entirely legitimate and are in no way reflective of your attachment to the baby. There is nothing wrong with asking someone to either return or temporarily store those items until you are more prepared to make some decisions. There is also nothing wrong if you decide to leave those items in place for the time being. Just know the decision should be based on what feels more helpful to *you*. Bottom line: Do not let anyone else decide how to handle your baby's belongings. You do not need any more surprises or loss of control.

Triggers Are Everywhere and Never-Ending

The real world is a very fertile world, and one that keeps turning even though yours feels as if it came to a complete stop. Pregnant women and babies will make for common sightings, and you likely will have some in your personal orbit as well.

The empty nursery, the minivan, and even a larger house that were all purchased to accommodate the expected addition now feel cruelly ironic. The triggers are inescapable: prepregnancy clothes that don't fit and maternity clothes that do, food and drink choices that were once off-limits are again available (even though you'd trade that glass of wine in a heartbeat to still be pregnant), and even the recommended continuation of your daily prenatal vitamin to help support you physically. These are daily reminders of a life that was supposed to have been but is not. The significant void in your world is all too obvious, and it hurts!

Bottom line: The triggers will continue to surround you and it's unrealistic that you (or anyone else) will be able to completely protect yourself from real life in the real world. Work to recognize and better accept this unfortunate and painful truth versus reacting in surprise every time you see or experience them. Be gentle and patient with yourself as you learn how to better navigate these sharp curves and work to take control to better buffer yourself where and when you can.

Common Example: The Baby Shower Invite

What You Can Do

Make individual and real-time choices based on how you're feeling, not based on what you think you should do. If you feel up to it, go. If not (for *any* reason), opt out and instead send a card, flowers, or a gift. It still can be hard to shop online for a baby gift for someone else, but that might end up being the lesser of two felt evils.

Sample Language

"It's honestly just too hard to see you pregnant right now. Our friendship is so important to me, but I need to step back and away temporarily to take care of myself. That is very hard to say, but I care enough about you to be honest. I can't ask that you understand, I just ask that you try. Please know I'm thinking of you and will reach out again when I can."

⸙ TRIGGERS AND SUPPORT GROUPS ⸙

Triggers can exist everywhere, even in believed safe places, such as a support group. Although such groups can be very valuable for some, for others, the risks and potential downsides may outweigh the anticipated benefits. Whereas the benefits include validation that you are not alone, and an increased sense of belonging and community (as well as access to additional perspectives and coping strategies at low or no cost), the downsides are real. There is an inherent expectation that you share your story, since the group works best if everyone participates. If you attend, you can anticipate being asked to share very personal and private information—something you may or may not feel ready to do. Further, you will be exposed to others' stories of loss and trauma, which, on one hand, can provide mutual support and empathy, but on the other hand, can also be something potentially upsetting and draining, especially when you are

(continues)

(continued)

already feeling quite compromised. You may do well to contact the group facil-
itator in advance to gather information about the current makeup of the group
so you both can better assess in advance whether it may be a good fit for you.

Taking Care of Yourself Physically

Whenever possible, rest, even if you cannot sleep. Try to eat healthier foods
and small snacks regularly throughout the day to keep a more constant and
controlled blood sugar level even if you don't have the appetite for full meals.
Keeping up your physical strength gives you a stronger base from which to
navigate all the emotional waves. Once you are medically cleared for exercise,
be active. Get outside and take a daily walk, breathing in fresh air and oxygen.
You can go back home and crawl into bed afterward, pulling the comforter
over your head, but take some deep, fresh breaths outdoors first. Watch your
alcohol and drug intake (including prescription medication). It's tempting to
try to numb yourself and escape the pain. However, that is only temporarily
and minimally helpful at best, and can often be hurtful and harmful if abused.
It can also further deepen your depressed mood.

Bottom line: Be smart about the choices you have and work to ensure you
are as physically healthy and grounded as possible.

⧼ YOUR PHYSICIAN CAN HELP ⧽

After a pregnancy ends (even prior to term), your body's sudden drop in hormones can trigger a strong emotional response. Ask your physician about
subsequent physical changes that may occur so you can best prepare for and
temper potential surprises or concerns.

If your loss just occurred (and you were sixteen to eighteen weeks' gestation
or later), discuss the potential for lactation, the option of milk bank donation
or ways to suppress milk production, and strategies to help reduce any physical

discomfort as the supply dries up. Clarify what you can anticipate about the return of your period as well as what that cycle may actually look like (for example, it may be heavier initially than it used to be). Most women experience a spontaneous return of menses four to eight weeks after their loss/surgery/delivery, with full-term losses falling on the latter end of that range. Becoming informed and knowledgeable about your body and the possible physical changes that can occur will help you care for yourself better during this time.

You may also consider talking with your physician about the option of medication, or asking for a referral to a psychiatrist to further discuss and address sleep difficulties and/or continuing symptoms of depression and anxiety. Medication may be helpful now *and even during a subsequent pregnancy.* Engage in conversation with a licensed and experienced professional who can assess your individual symptoms and recommend the best options for support.

YOUR PARTNER

It is common you and your partner will have different reactions at rock bottom. The loss of a pregnancy or the death of a baby are two things that affect a couple at exactly the same time. In general, life circumstances, such as the death of a parent or loss of a job, tend to affect one person more than the other. In this case, you are *both* hurting and in need of support, and thus may be unable to give the other what you're used to giving—particularly at a time when both of you may be looking for those things the most. Although you may be used to operating as one, that does not apply to grief. Reactions to grief are highly individual, unpredictable, and can be inconsistent. Your partner may shut down emotionally or become stoic. He or she may share similar emotions or even grieve more deeply. Women tend to be more outwardly visible with their grief, needing to talk and cry more frequently and for longer periods of time. Men, however, are usually more concrete and may be better able to shift their focus to work or activities for which they feel needed, useful, and productive.

Talking with Your Partner About the Loss

This contrast in dealing with grief can create extraordinary stress between both people, as well as misunderstandings and hurt feelings. It can result in one person feeling behind, not as far along in their grief, and certainly more alone. It can also result in one person feeling bad or guilty for just being honest about being in a different place. Silently comparing and analyzing your grief won't help either of you in any way. Instead, it's important to talk about your inevitable differences as you both work to better accept them.

Common Example: "I'm still really sad and think about what happened all the time. Why don't you talk about it anymore?"

What You Can Do

Acknowledge what (and how) you're feeling, and that the other person may have a different reaction altogether. Clearly state your needs and preferences while also being sensitive to your partner's.

Sample Language

"I feel like you're losing patience with me. I know it's frustrating for you to listen to me repeat myself about how upset I am. You've told me it makes you feel helpless because you can't say anything that changes how sad I am. However, I still need to feel connected to you and that we are together in this. It helps when you simply put your arms around me and hold me tight. I don't have to keep talking in those moments. Maybe we can just be."

Or,

"It is helpful for me to be at work and have some sense of normalcy. That doesn't mean that I'm not sad, and it certainly doesn't mean that I don't care. I just can't change the past and it's hard for me to keep replaying it over and over. I don't want to do that because it only makes me feel worse. And really angry. I'll keep working to express my feelings to you because I realize that may make you feel less alone versus seeing me come and go to work or with friends seemingly unfazed."

Keep listening and talking about your different reactions, thoughts, feelings, needs, and preferences.

Bottom line: Don't make assumptions or expect your partner will experience everything as you do or feel everything that you feel when you feel it. That's entirely unrealistic. Work to tolerate your differences and accept them, even if you don't understand or agree with all your partner's reactions.

Contrary to the belief of many, marriages and partnerships do not necessarily fracture and end from the weight of grief. If divorce does occur, it's more likely due to preexisting issues the loss only brought closer to the surface. Relationships are tried and tested through grief, and the challenges faced can feel more exaggerated. By sharing and talking through feelings gently and honestly—and without judgment—your relationship can weather differing emotions and experiences.

AMANDA

Those first days, weeks, months were excruciating. I did my best to keep talking out loud, sometimes shouting, sometimes weeping, while I trudged through my grief. I was working through it and letting everyone around me know I was. I didn't care if I offended anyone. I educated those that needed to be educated. I reached out to those who were too afraid to reach out to me because they didn't know what to say. My husband was not so verbal about his grief and there was a lot of conflict and frustration between us because of that. One very important thing I learned was that every person, no matter the sex, grieves differently. And it's not some linear timeline that you follow. It's ALL OVER THE PLACE. The grief and pain of losing a child never leave you. You never "get over it," but you do eventually learn to live with this new normal.

IF YOU HAVE OTHER CHILDREN

It is natural to want to protect your children from the pains of this world, but when life-changing events occur that acutely affect a family, it affects *the entire family*, regardless of age. Pretending that nothing has happened, or avoiding the conversation altogether, is not healthy for anyone.

Talking with Children About Loss

Death is a part of life, and it's important to use accurate and appropriate language with children so they can learn how to understand and then process it. Most mental health providers agree that children can understand the concept and permanency of death around age seven. However, even if they are too young to understand, they are intuitive and will pick up that something is different (including *your* being different). Most parents admit feeling awkward and ill-equipped to share the news of their loss with other children at home. They are still reeling from the tragedy, and worried they're somehow going to say the "wrong" thing. You can't and you won't if you're honest and heartfelt. But here's a guide to help you get started. Try to:

- **Keep it simple.** Being honest does not mean disclosing every single detail. You can simply state, *"The baby died."* or *"We're not going to have a baby anymore."*
- **Avoid euphemisms.** These could include *"The baby went to sleep"* as that could cause some children to begin to fear bedtime, worried something might happen to them, too.
- **Go slow. Pause. Assess the reaction.** Be prepared for a variability in response from sadness and tears, silence, to a desire to just go right back to play.
- **Validate the emotions and support what is expressed.** *"I know you are upset. You wanted a little brother or sister, and I wanted that for you, too."*
- **Avoid forcing a big conversation.** Children are adept at letting parents know what they need and when they need it. Questions will surface as children have them, not by your drawing them out. Some children may not ask any questions at all, and that's okay. Keep the lines of communication open. *"If you change your mind and have questions later, I want you to know you can always come to me. I will do my best to answer any questions you may have."*

Many parents may still feel apprehensive, concerned they are not prepared for every question they might be asked. Avoid that pressure. It's unrealistic for you to be able to anticipate every question, or always have a complete answer.

Keep in mind:

- You may be asked, *"Why?"* or *"What happened?"* If you have more information, again, be honest, and be sure to use age-appropriate explanations. (Your obstetrician and/or pediatrician can help guide you and suggest appropriate language or explanations.) For example, if the known cause of death was cardiomyopathy, you could say, *"The baby died. He had a rare disease that didn't allow his heart muscle to work like yours and mine."* Reinforce that you, your partner, and any other siblings are healthy and well. Give extra hugs to demonstrate your love and presence.
- It's always okay to say, *"I don't know. I wish I had an answer."* or *"I need to think more before I answer that. We can talk again later."* Then be sure to follow through.

Even though you may be focused mostly on your other children's emotions, don't forget to check in with your own.

How to Handle *Your* Emotions:
- Always be honest and heartfelt. Many parents create more stress and anxiety for themselves by working hard to keep their emotions in check, hidden even, concerned they're somehow going to damage their child if they're not holding it together emotionally. Remove the pressure of having to be someone you're not right now. There is nothing wrong (and everything right) with allowing your child to see your honest reactions (within reason), *even if that includes some tears.* (However, if you are crying hysterically, that can be scary and confusing and best expressed in private.) Again, children are intuitive. It is understandable and reasonable that you could become tearful and choked up when you tell your child, *"We're not going to have a baby anymore. And that makes me very sad."* In this case, your emotional reactions are consistent with your words, and that will make sense to a child, no matter the age. You're supporting yourself and your child's emotional development by sending the message that when someone is upset, it's okay to feel it, express it, and

share it. *"You know how much it hurts when you fall and scrape your knee and cry? Well, I hurt inside right now. I'm going to be okay, but for right now, I'm sad. I love you, and I'm so happy and grateful for you, even though I'm sad inside too."*

- Take a break. Pause the conversation if you begin to feel overwhelmed. It could be too much for *both* of you. You can always come back to it at a later time. *"Before we talk more, I need a break for a little bit. This doesn't mean I don't want to talk with you, it just means this is hard for me, and a cuddle might be better right now."*

Caring for Your Other Children

It is important to connect with your other children; however, you may feel emotionally ill-equipped at times, even uninterested, and with little to give. This isn't about what others think you should be doing, or expect you to be doing. It's about your obligation and responsibility to the children you have at home to ensure they are cared for properly and not create insecurity and anxiety for them, particularly those old enough to be aware of what is happening.

If you feel able, maintain your primary parenting role. If not, call upon your partner, a parent, sibling, or trusted friend to step in when you need time, space, and privacy to grieve. Recognize that you may feel guilty whether you force yourself to parent when you are emotionally compromised and unable to do so well, or if you delegate that task to someone else. Feelings of guilt are going to be present for a while (and not only in relation to parenting responsibilities). Work to be gentler with yourself and do your best to avoid self-judgment. The focus should be ensuring your other children's basic needs are met, whether you do the best you can in that moment or you delegate the role to someone else. Avoid making comparisons between how your children were cared for before and how they are temporarily being cared for now.

OTHERS' REACTIONS TO YOUR LOSS

There can be great and unexpected variability; in general, others' responses to grief and loss usually fall into one of three categories:

1. Honest, unassuming, and thoughtful responses that acknowledge inevitable limitations (for example, *"I'm so sorry. I can't find words that could or would necessarily provide comfort. But I'm here and want to support you in any and every way I can—by listening or talking, or giving you space and privacy."*). These types of responses are ideal because assumptions are not made about how (or what) you are feeling, and they do not superimpose or project their feelings and perspectives onto you.

2. Suggestive and interpretative responses from others (for example, *"Don't worry, you'll be able to have another baby."*). This not only suggests the false message that children are replaceable, but also a guarantee of success—neither of which should be expressed to any bereaved woman. Pregnancy is not a promise, and you have already learned that harsh lesson all too well.

3. Silence. No response, no acknowledgment of the loss (initially, but longitudinally as well). This reaction usually stems from awkwardness, personal discomfort with grief, or a desire to avoid saying or doing anything that will make you feel worse. It can also be an effort to better respect your privacy, intentionally avoiding discussing the loss unless you initiate. Unfortunately, for many women, that silence can be misinterpreted as a lack of care/concern.

⨳ YOU CAN TAKE CHARGE AND RESUME THE LEAD ⨳

It's likely you have already experienced some of what has been discussed and it can be challenging to field such unpredictable and variable reactions, especially now when you're feeling so fragile. But independent of others' reactions, you're not obligated to follow their lead. Instead, you can always redirect and inform others of the things most helpful to you. To help disengage: *"Please respect my/ our privacy. If and when it's helpful to talk more, I'll let you know."* Alternatively, to help engage: *"We haven't talked since I let you know we lost the baby. You probably don't know exactly what to do or say, but our relationship is very important to me, and I wanted to let you know it's beneficial for me to keep talking, and finding people who are willing to listen."*

What is curious is that people can and do surprise. The people you expect to stand up, step up, or show up, may not, while others may come out of nowhere and overwhelm you with their unexpected sincerity and thoughtfulness.

ANDREA

What do I wish people had said? What would I say? I wish I knew. I think each of us faces the journey in an astronomically personal way. I hope I would listen and not judge. I hope I would not apply my own experience. I hope I would react in a way that segregates the journey from the result. It is easy to connect them, but they are not connected. Mostly I hope there isn't anyone else in the universe who is going through what I did. If only.

My favorite response from a friend was a $5 Starbucks gift card. With almost no commentary, just a simple gesture that could evolve into a chat over some tea, a few moments alone with hot cocoa, or even just something warm to wrap my hands around on my way to work. She found an amazing way to show me that she just wanted to give me whatever I needed.

Many people are not going to know what to say or do with you. Some may remain inappropriately curious, bombarding you with questions and wanting to be very involved. Others may look at you with sad eyes or tiptoe around you, and if they do speak, it's only in hushed tones. Some may say nothing at all. It's important for you to be honest and express yourself in a way that is consistent with your emotions.

Bottom line: As you feel able, keep educating others on what is and what is not helpful to *you* at any given time. There is a greater chance your needs and preferences will be met if they are made known. Remember, grief is highly individual. There will be times when you will prefer space and privacy over company and community. For some, decreased social interaction, even intentional avoidance of others, can provide some relief. For others, being alone can feel like torture. Tune in to your feelings and do what is most useful for you. Your grief is going to be here for a while, and it's important that others can support you in ways that will be most helpful.

YOUR THOUGHTS MAY TERRIFY YOU BUT ALSO GUIDE YOU

At times, you may feel completely paralyzed at rock bottom, literally unable to move. But your thoughts still surround you. You will continue to grieve, but you might still focus on your decision and continuing desire for a baby and a family. These things haven't changed and your loss may have further solidified and even increased your desire for them. No future pregnancy or baby will ever replace or make up for the one you lost, but that is not the goal. You still desperately want to create your family. But where do you go from here? What does that look like, and more important, how do you get there? Especially, without a guarantee that you will conceive easily and when you desire. A guarantee you will have a routine pregnancy that results in the healthy, full-term delivery of a baby you can bring home and cherish. That's a lot to imagine, but it's likely where your thoughts are focused.

You are not alone. *Every* woman questions her path and doubts herself (and everyone around her) after losing her pregnancy or baby, certain she'll never be able to navigate ALL of the known hurdles ahead. Yet, it's important to realize that you can unintentionally make that path *impossible* by piling all the individual hurdles you may encounter ahead into one giant vertical stack. That sized hurdle is entirely unrealistic to leap, even for an Olympic athlete!

Trying to figure out all the answers *and* next steps *and* exact path *and* time frames *and* outcomes will only create more anxiety for you, and ultimately more frustration. Instead, focus on the one next hurdle, the one immediately in front of you. That's the hurdle of your grief. It's first because it's here, and it's here to stay for a while. It's not going to go away tomorrow, or next week, or next month. It's going to live with you for a long time. The challenge of this first hurdle is not for you to "get over it," it's for you to find a way to learn to live with it. No matter how much you wish it away or even wish to accelerate through it, there is no such thing as cutting corners with grief. It is hard and rigid and moves entirely at its own pace. That is the reality of grief.

As terrible as it is, your grief is your connection with your experience of pregnancy, your dreams for, and your memories of your precious baby. Today, those sacred memories can feel buried under the tragedy and the trauma of what you have experienced, and all you can touch are raw feelings. The first hurdle involves finding a way to acknowledge your grief and then better tolerate *and accept* a situation that was *completely and entirely* outside of your control to predict, to prevent, to direct, or to change.

Your grief will continue to be felt in every fiber of your being, but working to shift to a perspective of a growing acceptance will serve a twofold purpose:

1. It will allow you to access the more positive memories of your pregnancy or your time with your baby because the grief won't overshadow them—it will merely coexist with them.
2. This new perspective will help free, rather than fight, a part of you that you may be able to recognize and know again.

Once upon a time, you wanted a baby, you wanted a family. Due to a cruel and ironic twist of fate, that was not meant to be. However, deep down, that want—that wish—did not die with the pregnancy and the baby. Right now, grief and fear may be completely covering it, but that desire is still there inside you.

There is no question, you were struck by lightning and were gravely injured. Of course, the sound of thunder will startle and scare you. Now, it may only take dark clouds gathering and just the hint of rain to cause panic and keep you inside.

Bottom line: Your grief is here, it's real, and it's terrifying. But it would be an even greater tragedy if you never ventured outside again and *two* lives were lost instead of one. There is so much ahead you would miss that you cannot see right now because the grief is blinding. But that makes it all the more necessary and vital to address.

Future Grief

> It is the type of grief
> that can swallow one whole—
> losing a child.
>
> As the promise
> slides away in a moment,
> leaving a hollow that
> cannot be filled
>
> One may seek wisdom
> from the man high on a mountain,
> Sage, though he is,
> there are no answers
>
> One may go to Hades and back
> trying to revive
> the lost future,
> it will not be restored
>
> The gnashing of teeth
> and fits of rage
> will not bring her back,
> there is only surrender.
>
> **—BRITTANY**

﹛ 2 ﹜

The Depth and Duration of Grief

FOR MOST LOSSES, TIME IS considered a friend and bereaved individuals are encouraged to find comfort in their memories of the deceased. However, in the case of reproductive losses or the death of a baby, there are far too few, if any, memories. Losses that occur at the earliest part of the life cycle tend to be afforded considerably less sympathy by others with many erroneously believing there wasn't, couldn't have been, enough time to establish any type of a real relationship. As you are fully aware, that couldn't be further from the truth. The depth of grief has nothing to do with the length of the established relationship; it is more reflective of the depth of the attachment—something highly individual and unique to each relationship. That attachment likely solidified on some level the moment you confirmed you were pregnant. It wasn't as if you just started dating someone and were exploring the *possibility* of a future; instead, that commitment was made long ago, and you were actively planning for the rest of your life, and the rest of this baby's life, as an intact family.

Perinatal losses as a whole tend not to be recognized or discussed publicly. Many grieving parents who are vulnerable unknowingly take their cues from society about what is expected and reasonable in terms of the depth and duration of their grief. Unfortunately, this is primarily based on a limited understanding of the grief process as society views it, and one that is derived from the experience of an adult death, not that of an unborn baby or infant.

Perhaps most well-known is Dr. Elisabeth Kübler-Ross's pivotal 1969 work, *On Death and Dying,* in which she suggests a five-stage model for grief that includes the following phases: denial, anger, bargaining, depression, and acceptance.[1] Although some contemporary providers within the mental health community have challenged this stage model as outdated and overly facile, our society continues to talk of such things as "closure," "resolution," or an eventual conclusion to the grief process. This contrasts the view of many bereaved parents who instead know that on some level, grief is lifelong and is more about integration.

ERIN

This theory about stages of grief implies that once past a certain stage that emotion is now in the past. It hasn't taken me long to realize how untrue this is. These feelings of depression, anger, longing, and guilt come and go. Every day is different. Some stay away longer than others before returning; they vary in intensity with each visit and sometimes they visit all at once. I know that there is no end to this grief process. Time does not heal all wounds. It has helped me find ways to better cope with life without my daughter, but this is not a wound that will ever heal. I will live the rest of my life without a piece of my heart.

SOCIAL NORMS FOLLOWING ADULT DEATH

There are social norms in place that often dictate the roles and responsibilities of the surviving individual and the roles and responsibilities of all the other family and friends who surround that person. We know to say, *"I'm so sorry for your loss."* We know to send a card or flowers, to bring a meal. We know there will usually be some type of service or memorial to recognize the deceased person's life and to facilitate a sense of community in the wake of loss. And once the card is sent, the flowers/meal delivered, and the respects paid, most return (and quickly at that) to their own lives. A widowed grandparent is usually remembered on major holidays and anniversaries, as is a friend's loss of a parent on Mother's Day or Father's Day, but the remembrances tend to rapidly diminish in frequency and sentiment as time passes—in the case of all losses. To the bereaved but surviving individual, however, the void left by the deceased loved one is still heartbreaking whether that loss continues to be acknowledged or not. Silence may become the norm, but that doesn't mean the pain of loss is any less, and it may exacerbate feelings of isolation.

Society's understanding and tolerance of mourning are limited since the depth and duration of an individual's grief generally outweigh and outlast others' sympathies, independent of the age of the deceased individual. Well-intentioned others may sincerely believe that time heals all wounds, but in reality, their patience, tolerance, and comfort level with death is finite, resulting in a mixed message to "hurry up and grieve." For the bereaved, contact and interactions with others can often be confusing and filled with these mixed messages, neither of which are helpful for obvious reasons. Unfortunately, these flaws are highlighted in the context of reproductive losses and the death of a baby.

PERINATAL LOSSES ARE DIFFERENT

Despite efforts to increase awareness and sensitivity, perinatal losses remain significantly misunderstood and minimized. Reproductive losses and the death of a baby are remarkably different than any other type of loss for various reasons:

- **They upset the natural order.** We can feel ill-equipped and unprepared to respond even when death occurs at the end of the life cycle, or when advance notice is available; for example, following a long and terminal illness. But pregnancies and babies are supposed to be associated with new beginnings and life, not final endings. These types of losses are even more jarring, horribly unfair, cruel, and just plain wrong.
- **They represent a type of double loss.** In the case of the loss of a pregnancy or the death of a baby, not only are you reeling from the loss of everything you had anticipated ahead into the future, but *also* struggling in the absence of many (or any) comforting memories from the *past*. Several ultrasound pictures are very different than the collective and

somewhat comforting memories of years and years of birthdays, anniversaries, and holidays shared and spent together.

- **There are no well-established social norms.** As a whole, people find the topic of death awkward and uncomfortable. This is compounded when the death involves a child or a baby. People don't know what to do, what to say, and often try to express their sympathies quickly to fulfill an obligation and return to a more comfortable state. Standard adages often used with adults (for example, *"He lived a long and very full life. I hope you find comfort in your memories."*) are inaccurate and inappropriate in this case. The suggested message that "time heals all wounds" simply does not, and will not, work; it's just too big of an ask. Further, there is not always a service or memorial following a perinatal loss, which may end up enabling avoidance of the situation. In some cases, parents may even need permission to start grieving to allow for the release and full expression of their feelings instead of working to somehow adjust or contain them to reflect the generally limited messaging they've received from society: *"You'll get over this."* As awkward and as uncomfortable as society feels about your loss, the reality is no one feels as badly as you.

- **TWO people are affected deeply and simultaneously, but not in the same way.** Everyone has known a widow or widower and vicariously considered the depth of sadness and loneliness he/she feels after the death of a spouse. While that is a tough road to journey alone, the path of *two* grieving adults after a perinatal loss can be just as lonely. In this case, you and your partner must navigate very individual reactions simultaneously. As you might have already experienced, sometimes it can be even lonelier being with someone who is in a different place emotionally and/or mentally, than the physical company suggests. This quickly emerges as a challenge because you can't force your partner to fully understand or share your individual experience. That can cause stress and strain when you're both living under the same roof, but have very different needs and wants as well as opposing views of the things that are helpful. There can be felt differences in the individual grief experience, but as a whole, couples are initially somewhat forced into joint and time-sensitive decision-making (for example, *"What are we going to tell our other child at home?"* *"Should our families come into town?"*). However, as the weeks and months pass, there is the potential for even greater divide and distance within the couple's relationship as each experiences his or her grief more deeply as the reality of loss sets further in. Women may isolate themselves more, frustrated and discouraged when partners grow increasingly weary of hearing how sad they are. It's not uncommon to feel yourself shutting down, and sometimes even off. Men may attempt to problem solve, but when that's not well received, they may increasingly focus on work and outside friendships that feel more normal and accepting of their participation and presence. This does not mean that the couple's relationship will end. It simply means that increased tolerance, patience, acknowledgement, and acceptance of inevitable differences are invaluable as both parties work to navigate their grief and identify the things that are helpful to each individually.

- **There is no replacing the deceased, and yet, total family size is still evolving.** When an immediate adult family member dies—for example, a parent—the finite family size is reduced by one. That parent will never be replaced. Perinatal losses can create some confusion when they occur in families who are still working to create their final size. Although you also cannot replace a deceased baby, you can consider having another baby and growing your family. Bereaved parents are understandably and appropriately sensitive to the idea of a *"replacement baby."* This concept is impossible to fathom because the truth is, NO ONE WILL EVER REPLACE YOUR BABY. However, you will soon be forced to confront (if you haven't already) your plan and desire for family growth. In spite of your pain, the emerging reality is you wanted a baby, you wanted a family. And, it's up to you if you're still going to act on that despite your grief. But, in so doing, others may misunderstand, believing that baby can and will somehow restore both you and your family.

TIME BECOMES THE ENEMY

Grief following a pregnancy loss or the death of a baby is undeniably over-whelming, and can even feel paralyzing, but added to that is the additional pressure of time. You may feel this from every direction—from everyone and everything outside of you, as well as from deep within yourself.

Hurry Up to Catch Up (to Yourself)

Whether admitted or not, like other grieving women, you may feel the inevi-table weight of self-imposed comparisons to both your anticipated experience of fertility and family growth, and that of the rest of the world's experiences and successes. During your reproductive years, you probably have devised a general life plan that includes the timing and estimates of when you ideally want to start a family, how many children you desire, and even the spacing of those children. Following a perinatal loss, and especially if you've experienced recurrent pregnancy losses, you're now acutely aware that these plans have gone awry, bringing with that an uncomfortable loss of control.

ERIN

Yet, somehow, comingled among the shock, guilt, longing, anger, and depres-sion, I also felt the need to get pregnant again. I felt like I was running out of time and if I didn't do it now, I would come to my senses and never try again. I felt the need to get back on track with the life I had before our daughter died and somehow thought it would bring me hope and make life bearable again.

The reality of limited time and the knowledge that you have been kicked off course may further spur a sense of urgency to try again sooner than later. Having been on the wrong side of the line once (or more than once), you may now be hypersensitive to the fear of a repeat loss. After all, you now know bet-ter than anyone that pregnancy is not a promise. And, that's assuming you can conceive again, a serious concern for any woman who has already had a less than straightforward path toward conception. If you have had fertility issues, you already know that intrauterine insemination (IUI) and in vitro fertilization (IVF) involve so much more than identifying the possible window of ovulation and having unprotected sex. These are processes that take time and energy, and are stressful—especially when you're already feeling that you're starting from behind the curve. Continuing grief reactions may be compounded and truncated because of this understandable sense of urgency.

MARNEY

I remember when we had talked to the doctor and she said that I needed at least 6 months to heal before we could transfer our frozen embryos. I remember lying in bed and just sobbing that it would be at least another year plus before we could possibly have another baby. The thought of that just blew me away . . . we had tried so hard to have our daughter and then we lost her. My son would run up and down the halls yelling, "Where is my baby sister?" I felt guilty on so many levels and the thought that we had to do this all over again was beyond words. I had lost all glimmers of hope that this was actually going to work for us.

Hurry Up to Catch Up (to the Rest of the World)

It seems as if pregnant women and babies exist *everywhere*. The signs of fertility are all around and procreation is ongoing, which can highlight your own perceived shortcomings and experienced failures. Although you may be hesitant and too embarrassed to admit it, you may even feel in active competition with others, always acutely aware of your position (and theirs) in the race to create, and then complete, your family.

For example, independent of the integrity of the established relationship, it can feel especially painful when a younger sibling conceives or delivers a baby before you. Sisters, sisters-in-law, next-door neighbors, coworkers, friends, and even your physician all can, and sometimes do, conceive before you do again.

It is not uncommon to feel strong stabs of jealousy, anger, and resentment toward other women/couples who conceive before you do, particularly if it is someone close to you. This experience can intensify your grief, making it feel further unfair and alienating. It can deepen the sense of injustice in your world, disrupt your sense of the right order of things, and compound your frustrations, especially if your friend's pregnancy was not as difficult as your own and if it didn't involve loss. These emerging feelings can be alarming and sometimes even include thoughts of actual ill will toward the pregnant woman. For example, "*I was shocked to find myself wishing she would have a miscarriage or that something bad would happen to her baby or her. Because maybe she'd start to get a sense of what I'm going through or, at the very least, not have everything handed to her without any seeming effort.*"

The pressure mounts as you realize the overwhelming majority of women can and do conceive straightforwardly. You are not only reminded of others' fertility with great regularity, but also of unintended conceptions. How does it make you feel when a friend or colleague states, "*We weren't even trying and we conceived!*" or you hear or read about teenage pregnancies where conception wasn't only unintended, but also unwanted?

Negative projection (or Freudian projection) is a defense mechanism unconsciously employed when difficult and undesirable feelings are directed or attributed to someone else versus openly addressing the unwanted and uncomfortable thoughts or feelings themselves.[2] You may find that you feel resentment and anger toward innocent others who take advantage of their own fertility. It can feel like a slight when others can and do conceive on their own time frames, and your reaction is, "*I can't believe she got pregnant NOW, when she knows how much I'm hurting!*"

This idea is well illustrated through work with my patient who I'd seen through years of unsuccessful fertility treatments. She had made the difficult decision to take time off from her pursuit of parenthood and proceed with a rest cycle, feeling utterly exhausted both physically and emotionally. Instead of immediately plunging back into the next IVF cycle after the most recent failed one, she and her husband had decided to go white-water rafting in an effort to find rest, relaxation, and privacy away from restaurants and resorts brimming with children and families.

As she and her husband were rafting the rapids, instead of feeling relaxed and peaceful, her eyes were distracted by two dragonflies that were hovering above her raft and following her downstream, mating in midair. In many areas of the world, the dragonfly is associated with transformation or self-realization, usually serving as a symbol of life change. My patient was immediately aware not of its spirit or symbolism, but of the natural yet crude visual of its mating. Here was a dragonfly, a small, stupid creature that was doing something every other living thing on the planet could do, yet she could not. How startling and how crushing that felt to see something else procreate so naturally, so easily, and so successfully, *right in front of her eyes*. She felt as if the insect was mocking her. Distracting. Hugely disappointing. Disheartening. Disgusting.

It is normal and natural for you to feel extreme hypersensitivity and hyperawareness of everyone else's fertility and family planning efforts. While on some level, your grief and trauma dramatically and instantly matured you beyond your years, you are still human and will continue to experience the full range of human emotion, including deep feelings of jealousy and even resentment toward others who have what you had and continue to want desperately. Most women are disappointed in themselves for making such unfair and unhelpful comparisons, but find it difficult to turn off that ongoing narrative. Further, many feel ashamed and even disgusted by themselves when their inner voices may condemn those who did not suffer through such a painful loss, and may even harbor dark thoughts about others, wishing their paths were somehow harder. These thoughts are not intentionally malicious, but instead, signs of the deep desperation of pain and loss, and not wanting to feel so alone, lost, and left behind. The emotional element here is enormous.

In some cultures, women define themselves by the ability to create life and become a parent, a mother. The less-than-straightforward path toward this end, and for many the great struggle, can create feelings of inadequacy, failure, and a corresponding (and profoundly negative) impact on a woman's sense of identity.

You may try to limit interactions and contacts, but, at some point, it becomes impossible to avoid, especially if you are asked to be a godmother to your younger sister's new baby or to help host a baby shower for your best friend. These interactions are complicated, and there is not always the desired sensitivity and understanding on the receiving end of why it can be so painful to be around someone else's growing belly, to hold someone else's newborn, or to be around someone else's young children. You can make an effort to educate others about your feelings, but education can be exhausting, and it's still not a guarantee they will understand the very complicated and complex emotions you might not always even understand yourself. Some relationships are strengthened by honest and open disclosures, but some might become forever changed, or even end. And so, the loss remains something outside of your control and only continues to widen and deepen with the passing of time, and everyone else's growing fertility successes.

Hurry Up and Grieve

You already know all too well that there is no such thing as "getting over it," even though others will have a limited ability to understand or have tolerance for your sadness over your loss. The challenge is learning how to live with the loss of your pregnancy or the death of your baby. However, no clear formula outlines exactly how to do this. Even with the knowledge that on some level grief is going to be ongoing as far as you can see, most women still pressure themselves to hurry it along, because grief feels just *awful*. It's dizzying and disorienting. It's messy and raw and unpredictable. The things that are both helpful and unhelpful can change rapidly and without notice. You may not even recognize yourself right now, but that doesn't stop you from desperately wishing you could find yourself, or anything that feels better or normal. But for many, the meaningful things that are "better" or "normal" (such as taking comfort in a living child at home) may be inaccessible immediately, or simply feel temporarily impossible.

ERIN

It would have made sense for me to be more drawn to my living son when my daughter died three weeks after birth, but it was the opposite. Every time I

looked at him, I saw what was missing and it took me a while to be able to be
a parent to him again.

Whereas some women can and do resume parenting responsibilities, for many, it's a much less straightforward process. And even in cases where a living child at home serves as a motivating force to get out of bed or get through daily activities, parenting still can require extraordinary effort.

Another reason that women may try to accelerate their grief is that the tasks of grieving and trying again are believed impossible if attempted simultaneously. And yet, the conception of another pregnancy honestly may be *the one and only* thing you can identify that gives you any hint of hope for happiness in your future.

ALLISON

I'm a physician and went back to work six days [after my loss]. Three weeks later . . . we were intimate again. I drank alcohol again for the first time, and I began to feel like a human being after living in a darkness that is hard to even remember now. But in that return of humanity, all I could do is feel an intense physical emptiness that I knew would only be filled with another pregnancy. There was really no decision of whether to try again. I did not feel guilty about wanting to replace the baby we lost—I felt like I would not survive emotionally or physically if I did not get pregnant again. I wanted to jump back into what I just unexpectedly was kicked out of. There was no moment of questioning whether I could handle it emotionally, it felt like my emotional health was dependent on being pregnant again.

As with all loss, acute grief reactions generally continue longer than most anticipate or expect. If you are finding yourself at this juncture, you are well aware that time is not a luxury you can afford. Most women quickly realize that if they waited until they felt 100 percent better or stronger before trying, they would never try again. The weight and worry can feel overwhelming as the mind wrestles with a multitude of questions and hard truths:

> *"What if I don't conceive as straightforwardly as before?"*
> *"What if I can't ever conceive again?"*
> *"What if there are complications?"*
> *"What if I have another loss?"*
> *"I was ready for a baby a long time ago and that didn't work out."*
> *"I'm so far behind where I had thought I'd be."*
> *"I feel so empty and overwhelmed."*
> *"I think the only thing that is going to even partially fulfill me is to be pregnant again."*

And so, it quickly emerges: You cannot and will not be able to outrun your grief. Your desire for another pregnancy is likely only increasing with each passing day. You are, therefore, going to have to figure out a way to tolerate both grieving and trying again simultaneously if you are going to grow your family.

Hurry Up and Say Yes

Those who have experienced a perinatal loss and decide to pursue another pregnancy must confront continuing grief, depression, anxiety, and sometimes trauma reactions. This is all against the backdrop of the simultaneous challenges of ever-advancing maternal age, increasing risks with the passing of time, and the unavoidable and rapidly closing window of reproductive opportunity. Under this kind of pressure, the traumatic injury is not allowed to begin to heal and scar over time, as is the case with other losses. Instead, this wound is forced to remain open and gaping as you face the inevitable question of *"Do I dare consider doing this again?"* But, even when you are able to navigate *all* of the above challenges, there remains yet one more: getting your partner on board and also ready to say yes.

SARAH

I think one of my doctors mentioned that we could have more children while we were still in the hospital. At the time it seemed preposterous, but the seed was planted. Over the next few weeks, we talked about it a little. Because of our ages (I was forty and my husband was forty-one), we knew that if we were to have more children, we didn't have a lot of time to think about it.

Despite historically acting as one, it is not uncommon for couples to have very different thoughts and feelings both about trying again and the timing in which to do so. When initiating conversation with your partner about trying again, you may be especially sensitive to your partner's reactions, looking for validation and reassurance of your perspective, but not always receiving the same back. (If you've experienced recurrent pregnancy loss, you may feel added pressure not only about your timing, but also your ability to get your partner back on board, concerned there are only a finite number of times he or she is going to say yes.) There may be times you want your partner's input, and there will be times you don't. You partner may legitimately express concern about the amount of suffering you have displayed since your loss and thus remain hesitant to engage in conversation about trying again, wanting to protect and shield you from the possibility of more loss. However, you may react to such a stance with anger, viewing it as offensive, punitive, and quite hurtful.

JACKIE

This is where things got really difficult, really crazy. We were at a complete loss. While grieving, I was still wondering what the next step could be, but dared not pursue any thoughts, any hope. I was terrified to discuss this with my husband thinking he would want to stop altogether and I knew that he was not in favor of adoption. Rather than moving ahead, I was in limbo and just trying to find some answers for many months—answers that never came, but it was the quest for them that proved important.

Despite you and your partner's overall increased sense of vulnerability, grief, fear, and stress, it is critical to keep communicating. *"Not now"* does not mean *"not ever."* *"I'm scared"* doesn't mean *"I won't."* By initiating the conversation about trying again, you are doing *something*. And, by doing something, you work to move time from the position of being the antagonist to becoming the ally.

CHASING TIME

Pregnancy and the pursuit of parenthood can easily be compared to a marathon. Women who are in the race feel a sense of community, and there is unlimited excitement and energy in the air with everyone focused on the finish line—the arrival of a healthy, full-term baby.

Tragically, at some point along the way, you experienced the loss of your pregnancy or baby, and were abruptly kicked out of the race you anticipated completing along with all the other registered runners. That unexpected and unwanted ending was—and is—excruciatingly painful, especially when you were so ready and prepared. It's one thing to lose after a fair race, but something altogether different when you were not even allowed the full run. And then, there is yet more loss—the loss of time. This loss is even deeper than is first apparent. Many women are temporarily frozen and unable to even walk back up to the start line to begin running again because just like preparation for a marathon, there is often more training required before the race can even be entered again. This "training" takes the form of waiting for an HCG (human chorionic gonadotropin) level to return to zero, waiting for the return of menses, being advised to wait three normal periods before trying again, waiting to begin medication in advance of another egg retrieval or transfer, waiting to test, realizing the latest attempt for conception was not successful, and so forth.

This analogy of a pregnancy being like a marathon (including the time and arduous training investment even before race entry) only underscores the cruel and painful steps you must retrace before beginning a race you thought you were already running. It's as if the announcer called every runner to her starting place as everyone waited and listened for the pistol shot to begin. This lone action and sound signaled the beginning of the last pregnancy . . . and the beginning of an expected future. But, at some point in your race, you received a sharp kick to the stomach and were ripped out of your place only to be violently thrown even further behind the original start line.

Yet, despite your injuries, your vision remained entirely intact and you were forced to watch as all the other runners continued in the race, running well, ever advancing... and then crossing the finish line to receive congratulations and celebrations. You, on the other hand, feel lost and overwhelmed in your acute grief as well as paralyzed, stuck in time, far behind, and wondering if you ever can or ever will catch up not only to the finish line, but even to the starting line. You may feel deeply impatient, so ready to get on with your life. But you know it's entirely outside your control and that time is running out... and it's running out *FAST*.

﹛ 3 ﹜

The Wait (and Weight) Surrounding When to Start Trying

EVEN WITH A BILLION UNANSWERED questions about how you will ever be able to survive another pregnancy, you may instinctively and definitively know that trying again *is* something you are going to do, but you may wrestle with thoughts about *when*.

You may feel ready to begin the process immediately (or that you *have* to—for example, if you've experienced recurrent pregnancy loss), and that you cannot become pregnant again soon enough. One reason for this is being acutely sensitive to the idea of "lost" time, wanting to take proactive measures to get back on course quickly. Conversely, you may not even be able to fathom that possibility for some time. Or, like many women, you may still be unsure and need time to weigh the many pros and cons of both waiting and not waiting before deciding. *All* these reactions are valid, and worthy of more consideration before that decision is finalized and then acted upon.

﹛ **JENNY**

I've always wanted to have a bigger family but have a lot of anxieties, guilt, etc., about being pregnant again. I think we probably will go for it, but I need

a little more time to process everything that's happened. I do expect that be-
ing pregnant again could be quite healing (despite all the nerves and emotions
that will come along with it). I know having a miscarriage would be devastat-
ing but so much less so than it seemed before the last month. Interesting how
your perspective and fears can change in such a short period of time. It feels
very strange/stupid/brave/disloyal to be thinking about this again. But I know
life goes on. Life moves forward. Decisions must be made. This is both a bless-
ing . . . and a curse.

Due to your obstetric history, and even after a careful and thorough decision-making process, it is highly likely you will continue to question and second-guess your decision about timing. You may feel this at various points during ongoing attempts for conception, and even while pregnant. This is not about the quality of your decision; rather, the weight of it. And, ultimately, it's also about fear. Again, you've long realized if you waited until you felt completely ready before jumping back in, you'd wait the rest of your life.

When you have experienced loss, your overall sense of self is injured, including your self-confidence. Taking a definitive and active stance to say *"I'm ready"* can feel like a big commitment, and the fear created by intentionally walking back into the fire after being severely burned can be immobilizing. Even though you know you desperately want what (and who) is potentially on the other side, preparing to walk over coals and through flames while you still have blistering burns is frightening. Although highly uncomfortable, indecision may feel like a safer alternative.

While you have *some* time, the reality is that you don't have *unlimited* time, so identifying and confronting your fears is paramount. You will feel better about yourself and your decision (and more in control) if you make an active decision versus a passive one (that is, waiting until time makes the decision for you).

The majority of women who experience perinatal loss (approximately 80%) will usually decide to try again *and conceive* within eighteen months.[1]

And, just like these women, you *can* determine a point at which you are willing to start trying again, even if you don't feel entirely ready as yet.

HOW DO I KNOW WHEN THE RIGHT TIME IS FOR *ME*?

For you to answer that question, you're going to need to gather information and have earnest conversations with:

1. Your physician
2. Your partner
3. Yourself

The conversations may occur simultaneously or sequentially. They are not listed in order of importance because all of these are essential. You may not like all the information you receive, but it's still necessary for you to engage with and reconcile all three perspectives.

What follows are necessary steps toward ensuring your decision is fully informed and medically sound, mutually agreed upon with your partner, and one in which you feel as comfortable and confident as possible.

TALKING WITH YOUR PHYSICIAN
First, Decide Whether to Stay or Go

You may find yourself with mixed feelings about your current physician. For example, you may be grateful for all the medical and emotional care received historically, but also anxious and questioning whether this is the right relationship and office for you going forward, given all the associations with your loss.

ERIN

Going back to the same OB's office for my six-week postdelivery checkup was awful. This is the same office that I sat in through two pregnancies as an excited expectant mother who was sure that nothing terrible could ever happen to her or her babies. Now I sat there as a mother who had given birth six weeks ago to a child who was no longer alive. It made me angry to see other blissfully naïve expectant mothers in the waiting room. I miss being that kind of mother. I realized that I would need a different doctor and waiting room to sit in with our subsequent pregnancy.

MARY

After experiencing two miscarriages and a prenatal diagnosis, we felt the next pregnancy would be difficult and anxious enough on its own, so we did not want to take on the stress of finding a new OB/GYN on top of that. It was comforting to know that our doctor knew our whole history so if (well, really when) I burst into tears or wasn't giddy at the first ultrasound, I wouldn't have to explain.

Carefully consider your current physician and overall office experience to date (including interactions with ancillary staff, wait/response time to questions, and requested scheduling) and either confirm the decision to stay or begin to explore the option of transferring care. There are pros and cons to both staying with your existing physician and to leaving. This is a highly personal decision, but it is vital that this also be an active decision and choice rather than a passive acceptance. No physician or office is perfect, but having the right rapport and comfort level with the staff you will be interacting with regularly will be critical in preparing and supporting you through the pregnancy ahead.

A search for a new physician can feel overwhelming, from seeking referrals, to the time spent determining who is accepting new patients and has a schedule that accommodates yours, to the emotional investment in meeting/interviewing that person, and reviewing your full (and sensitive) obstetric history. Or it may feel like a relief to avoid returning to an office where the physical space alone could trigger painful memories (for example, an exam room where you received bad news).

Choosing to transfer care doesn't have to be a reflection of the relationship or care previously provided. It can simply reflect a need for a different environment or experience that isn't associated with loss. Selecting the right person and office to serve your current medical *and* emotional needs are well worth the time and effort spent. Regardless of whether you remain with your current physician or pursue a transfer of care, it is in your best interest to begin the following medical conversations now.

๕ THE CASE OF THE PREGNANT PHYSICIAN ๑

Many female physicians are of childbearing age. If you discover that your OB/GYN is pregnant and that causes you any discomfort, express your feelings and concerns directly. Sample language might include, *"I'm very sensitive to others' pregnancies right now. I'd like to ask for a referral to another physician as I think your pregnancy could be uncomfortable and distracting for me, and potentially disruptive in my care."* Your physician should be willing and able to refer you to another provider. By being proactive, you will avoid further awkwardness or discomfort.

Be Vocal and Direct About Your Interest in a Subsequent Pregnancy

Most women who experience loss *immediately* begin thinking about a subsequent pregnancy, but are also hesitant or afraid to ask about timing, believing their physician will somehow think they are being inappropriate and premature under the circumstances. If you don't ask, however, there's a chance of further delay.

The conversations held with patients at the time of loss vary greatly. Some physicians will initiate a discussion about the possibility and timing of a subsequent pregnancy as part of their loss conversation with you, wanting to empower and educate you should you wish to become pregnant again. Out of respect for your grief, other physicians will avoid the topic and wait for you to initiate the discussion. However, *all* physicians are willing to have this conversation and can provide valuable medical guidance as to when you can safely and actively begin attempts for another pregnancy.

QUINN

And there I sat. In the hospital with the neonatologist and my husband by my sides. Both were talking to me and trying to kindly and lovingly support me after we had just lost our son, six weeks after delivery. I was devastated, destroyed, and crying over our dead baby. They both actually looked kind of afraid of me in that moment because I was a complete mess. But neither realized everything going on in my head and my heart. I was also crying about my future. I wanted to be a mom, but because my son died, I didn't get to be a mom. I was afraid to ask about another pregnancy because I knew then they'd think I was crazy for real. I mean, who sits there with a dead baby in their arms, sobbing over losing him but at the same time trying to find a way to ask about creating another? Even with a broken heart, I knew I still really, Really, REALLY, wanted to be a MOM.

Determine the Specific Medical Advantages or Disadvantages Behind Any Recommended Wait

Have a thorough and in-depth conversation with your physician about the timing of trying again. In the event you are quickly cleared and given a medical green light, avoid any self-imposed pressure to begin immediately. Instead, continue to explore the psychological and emotional aspects of your decision about timing. (Experienced mental health providers can also give a useful perspective and extend valuable support as you work to navigate these influences.)

If there are any potential medical contraindications to your trying, it's important to identify and understand them *now* and to follow the medical advice closely to ensure your body is in the best possible condition to support another pregnancy.

Historically, after a loss, most physicians counseled their patients to wait three months before trying again. That was before ultrasound was used to establish an accurate due date. Now, most physicians agree that after an early first-trimester loss, most women should wait one normal menstrual cycle before trying again. For later losses, physicians may recommend waiting anywhere from three months to as long as twelve to eighteen months, particularly if the loss occurred at term.

No matter what time frame is suggested, it can be helpful for you to:

1. Confirm that your physician's recommendation is exclusively a medical rather than a *combined* medical/emotional recommendation. Right now, you are only looking to clarify with your physician what is best and safest for your body.
2. Make sure you fully understand the exact reasons behind any medically advised wait. Don't hesitate to ask questions for clarity. Although any recommended delay can be difficult to accept emotionally, a complete intellectual understanding of it will help you endure a wait of any length.

Discuss Other Possible Influences That May Affect Timing

After a loss, many patients consent to additional testing (for example, maternal blood work, surgical/placental pathology studies, and/or autopsy), hoping it will yield some clues or answers as to what went wrong, as well as help inform a future pregnancy. Know it is normal to experience strong emotional reactions regardless of what results are returned.

You may become upset in the event something is identified, or a condition or disease is diagnosed. Even with a clear and identifiable cause of death, and concrete information that can be useful for the next pregnancy, it can be hard to accept the fact that "*There was something wrong with my baby.*" Also, if you pursued an autopsy and the final report was returned inconclusive, there can be equally deep upset and even more fear, as you are left without something identifiable to target and work to prevent the next time.

Discuss and weigh the possibility of obtaining new information against the closing window of time. It is common to want to wait to begin trying again until all final reports are obtained, something that could take weeks or months. Depending on your age, your physician may advise you that waiting will negatively impact your chances for conception. You may also be unprepared for the level of disappointment, sadness, and frustration you experience if you miss a potential window of ovulation or the next IVF cycle because you are waiting on test results, especially if those results are later returned inconclusive. This doesn't mean you shouldn't look for answers; it means you should be prepared for the possibility you may not find them.

Lastly, although the medical recommendations for interpregnancy intervals tend to be consistent among physicians overall and based on the body's physical needs, several other factors may influence *your* sense of timing. They include your age, the total number of children you desire, and your preferred spacing of those children. Acknowledge these factors and share them with your physician. He/she can also provide valuable counsel and perspective about what is medically safest for you.

Consider and Discuss the Pros and Cons of Seeking Out a Specialty Consultation

Even with a return to physical baseline (resumed menses) and medical clearance, most bereaved women remain hesitant to completely trust their bodies to do this again and worry that they or their primary physician may have missed something. Most women turn to the internet, actively searching for more information and answers, and chasing a desperate desire for any sense of reassurance and control. And many women consider seeking the same from an independent specialist (if one is available in their geographic area), such as a reproductive endocrinologist (RE), or maternal-fetal medicine (MFM) physician.

Reproductive endocrinologists are board-certified physicians who first train as OB/GYNs. These physicians have received additional training in reproductive medicine and address hormonal functioning as it pertains to reproduction, as well as the issue of infertility. For reference and within the general population, a referral to a reproductive endocrinologist would be considered if any of the following criteria were met:

- You have been trying for conception without success for one full year.
- You are thirty-five years or older and considered advanced maternal age (AMA).
- Your menstrual cycles are irregular or have ceased.

- You have (or have a history of) a maternal or paternal reproductive condition (for example, endometriosis, PCOS, PID).
- You have a history of miscarriage or infertility.

Note, even with these generally agreed upon criteria, there is inconsistency and variability within the medical community as to when patients are referred. Some practices are very quick to refer; others don't refer out when they should. Some physicians would not refer their patient to a RE based on age alone and some would typically refer after *recurrent* miscarriage, but rarely after one.

Maternal-fetal medicine specialists are also board-certified physicians who have completed additional education and intensive training beyond their four years of OB/GYN training. These high-risk pregnancy experts provide care in the event something threatens the health or life of the mother, or her fetus. More specifically, a referral would be considered if:

- You have an existing medical condition (such as high blood pressure, obesity, diabetes, etc.).
- You experienced complications from a previous pregnancy (for example, preterm birth, preeclampsia, intrauterine growth restriction).
- There are health complications with the baby.
- You have a multiple gestation pregnancy (twins, triplets, or higher-order multiples), although many OB/GYNs oversee twin pregnancies without MFM involvement.

Two common misconceptions are that MFM care is indicated if a woman is thirty-five years of age or older (AMA), or if she has a history of loss (yet no other issues as just outlined). Neither of these factors alone suggests your next pregnancy will be high risk, or that you necessarily need to consult such a specialist.

You do not need a referral from your physician to schedule either of these consultations, but it may help to disclose your interest or intent to him/her if you are considering an appointment with either type of specialty provider. By doing so, you will better understand your physician's position and perspective on any anticipated benefits for you, and determine the level of potential collaboration. If your physician supports the idea, he or she might recommend an appropriate and trusted specialist for you to contact.

In the event your primary physician does not believe such a referral is medically indicated, *you* may still feel it necessary to explore due to maternal anxiety alone—wanting and working to check every single box you can find. If you decide you must see a specialist, be thoughtful and honest with yourself, clarify your specific intentions, and identify realistic expectations. Don't schedule the appointment just to feel like you're doing something. Instead, a visit to a specialist can be useful if:

- You meet medical criteria as determined by the particular specialty.
- You want the opportunity to review your loss history from an outside perspective and explore possible implications for conception and/or a subsequent pregnancy.
- You acknowledge (to yourself and the specialist) that your primary physician has already deemed you healthy and your body to be functioning normally, yet you are looking for a second opinion to reaffirm.

Recognize, however, even with a specialty consultation, you may *still* remain afraid as you continue steps toward a subsequent pregnancy. Not because you have somehow missed a box, but because you don't have the one thing that could reduce that fear: a guarantee that this time will be different.

MARNEY

To try again was never a discussion point for us. It was just something that we knew we were going to do. It wasn't a question of "if," it was a question of "when." Due to our fertility issues in conceiving our [deceased] daughter, we knew that we would need it [assistance] again for our future pregnancy. So, we immediately made an appointment to talk things out with our fertility doctor. We talked about what may have gone wrong, what can be done in the future, the timeline and what we needed to do for ourselves physically and mentally to

be prepared for the transfer of our two remaining frozen embryos. The transfer
would be in six months.

Leaving the doctor, she told us, "Lightning never strikes twice." I remember
being so disturbed by this statement because I thought that losing our baby
was so much worse than a lightning strike! And, I knew no one could really pro-
tect us from lightning ever striking again. I desperately wanted that guarantee,
but I knew no one could give me that.

Ironically, that statement continued to resonate through my mind over the
upcoming months and became somewhat of a mantra that would keep me
going in times of desperation.

⸲ RECURRENT PREGNANCY LOSS ⸱

Until recently, recurrent pregnancy loss (RPL) was defined as a condition whereby a woman experienced three or more clinical pregnancy losses before twenty weeks' gestation,[2] and physicians routinely referred patients who met these criteria to specialists. Even though the American Society for Reproductive Medicine (ASRM) recently redefined this term as *two or more* pregnancy losses, some physicians will still wait to discuss a specialty consult until you've had three losses. You may not be willing to wait for another loss and decide to self-refer to a specialist sooner. This is not uncommon, but recognize that physicians may have differing opinions about a referral at that point.

Find the Right Patient/Physician Balance

Relationships involve two people, and in this case, your role is that of the patient. You will need to find an appropriate balance between being a strong self-advocate and a well-informed follower. Do your best to process all medical information and recommendations. When you don't understand, or feel uncertain, *ask*. Ask again (and again) if you still don't. As you step further into this next pregnancy, you will probably feel increasing nervousness and fear. That's to be expected. The slightest hint of anything being "off" or any deviation from what you believe to be normal may cause you to spiral with extraordinary worry and the belief that something is horribly wrong. That's not necessarily the case, and you trying to play two roles simultaneously—that of patient *and* physician—will only create more stress. Instead, talk (and then listen) to your physician and address your concerns and fears together.

Maintaining open lines of communication with your physician is critical in building a stronger relationship and foundation of trust for managing a subsequent pregnancy. You still might not completely trust your physician after all you've been through, but ultimately, you may wind up trusting him/her more than you trust yourself and your body at this point.

By following these recommendations, you will be able to determine whether there are any medical advantages (or disadvantages) to waiting to try again. In the event there are identified medical benefits to waiting, it is wise to follow that advice to ensure your body is in the best physical condition possible to support another pregnancy, even if waiting feels frustrating and emotionally impossible. Although you may feel deeply sensitive to the great disappointment and additional loss of control, gaining knowledge, clarity, and understanding of the reasons behind the recommended wait may make the weight somehow more bearable.

TALKING WITH YOUR PARTNER

It is common to feel hesitant initiating a conversation with your partner about trying to conceive again. In fact, your partner may also feel reluctant to start a conversation with you. The main reason is that you *both* may be scared of finding out that you're not on the same page—and then what? But that's not a good reason to avoid the conversation. That fear is actually a strong reason to begin it. If you find you're both willing to consider another pregnancy and have similar ideas about timing, fantastic. Two hurdles crossed. However, if you find you're not on the same page, identifying that sooner rather than later will give you the time you need to explore and process your individual thoughts and feelings, and then work to find common ground on which you can both stand.

If you can't, couples therapy can be beneficial. Tiptoeing around the conversation, or avoiding it altogether, only results in more lost time.

How to Start:

- **Initiate conversation gently and respectfully.** Instead of leading with *"We have to talk"* (which can put anyone on the immediate defense), consider how you ideally prefer to be approached, and also how your partner best receives requests and information. Lead in a more unassuming way such as saying, *"Would you please help me?"* Also consider the positive impact of lowered volume, or a slower rate of speech. Both can be calming and encourage more active listening.

- **Avoid making assumptions about what your partner is thinking or feeling.** This should be obvious, but we all can benefit from the reminder.

- **Use "I" statements and simple terms to express what you are feeling.** Consider something like *"I'm feeling anxious,"* *"I'm struggling,"* or *"I feel alone."*

- **Identify how your partner can help, and be open to ways you might return that favor.** Instead of immediately jumping in, first be specific about your partner's requested role—do you want a listener, a problem-solver, etc. *"It's not so important that you necessarily agree with all of my thoughts and feelings, but it is important that you listen. I'd like you to hear where I'm at."* You can add, *"I'm also hoping to learn more about what you're thinking/feeling, and how I can best support you. Even if we're not exactly on the same page, I'd like to keep working in that direction together."*

- **Be strategic and sensitive about timing.** Don't assume that just because you're ready to talk before bedtime or in the first quiet opportunity of the day, that your partner feels the same. He or she might be exhausted and just wanting to rest. Be considerate and find a day/time that work for you both: *"I recognize there's a lot to cover, and to make it less overwhelming, perhaps we could start by carving out 30 minutes sometime tomorrow and then agree to another time to continue talking this weekend."*

- **Express gratitude.** These conversations can be difficult for you both. Even if you don't make the desired progress you want or expect immediately, recognize that just starting the conversation is forward movement. Thank your partner for being willing and able to listen—that is a true gift.

When talking with your partner about trying again, you may be especially sensitive to his or her reactions, looking for validation and reassurance of your perspective, but not always receiving it. There may be times when you want your partner's input and times you don't, especially when the opinion or perspective differs from yours. And, in some cases, your partner's response may even create pressure, particularly if he or she defers to you about the timing of trying again, by saying, *"It's your body, and there's so much more you have to go through. I'll do whatever feels best/right for you and be ready whenever you are ready."*

Although these types of statements are intended to be kind, they can unintentionally put more pressure on you to shoulder the entire weight of the decision yourself when you are already feeling compromised emotionally and psychologically, and sometimes physically as well. You may also pressure yourself to act stronger and more confident than you actually are for fear of having the decision delayed or taken away from you. You may think: *"If my husband really knew how sad I was, he would absolutely question my readiness to have another child."*

Your partner may legitimately be cautious about jumping back in, still grieving the recent loss, but also feeling that, on some level, he or she has lost a part of *you*, too, and unwilling to risk losing more. Any hint or suggestion of hesitation or delay can be hard to hear, but it's important for you to know how and what your partner is feeling, just as your partner needs to know how and what you're feeling. This perspective is not a criticism, not a judgment, and not a reason for you to mask your true feelings and emotional state to secure the green light from your partner now. You are both grieving and doing the best you can, but your individual needs may be different. It's crucial to acknowledge and work through that to get to a place where you can both exist.

ROBYN

We decided to meet with a high-risk [maternal-fetal medicine] practice about four months after our loss. Although in some ways it felt early, I needed to know what our options were. To our surprise, the physician was supportive of another pregnancy. A month later, we met with another practice to get a second opinion, and that physician was supportive as well. The reality is that it wouldn't matter how many medical opinions we get because my husband is terrified about another pregnancy. How could he not be scared? As scared as I am as well, I am even more terrified of living my life with major regret.

Instead of avoiding your differences, continue to talk about them. Be honest. Listen to each other. "*I'm scared*" does not mean "*I'm never going to be willing to try this again.*" It simply means "*I'm scared.*" Challenge yourself to find words that express what you really mean. If you continue to work as you have been for the duration of your relationship—not as members of the opposition, but as a team—you can and will achieve unity. With teams, everyone has a different role and position. In the huddle, the forward may greatly benefit from the goal tender's perspective of the plays already completed, and those that should be considered at the start of the next period. Even if the forward is very sure of the next play, the goal tender's vantage point and perspective are invaluable. The team is strengthened as a sum of the individuals, each of whom carries his or her own views and ideas but finds ways to, ultimately, work as one.

RESUMING SEXUAL ACTIVITY

When it comes to resuming sex after a loss, couples and individuals vary considerably. Even before you are medically cleared to be sexually active again, you may find yourself desiring sex for the emotional intimacy aspect alone. Or you may find you initially have no interest in physical intimacy or sex *at all*.

(continues)

(continued)

Grief and trauma often blunt positive feelings, including sexual desire. Wherever you find yourself on the spectrum, talk openly and honestly with your partner to express your thoughts, feelings, and expectations. Silence has a way of being misunderstood, and assumptions can be made that can create distance at a time when you're focused on getting ready to work together again. Rather than leaving your partner in the dark, summon the courage to express your true feelings, and ask for patience if you need more time. Whenever you do decide you're ready, remember, there's the potential of conception occurring *before* your period returns. Conceiving before you are medically cleared can set you up for more heartache and lost time in the event your body is not yet able to physically support another pregnancy and ends in another loss. If you determine you are going to wait, proactively discuss birth control and then be diligent about using it.

INVOLVING FAMILY/FRIENDS/OTHERS IN THE CONVERSATION

As with any big decision, it is common to want to talk about it with family and close friends. But the solicited—and unsolicited—advice from those closest to you is not always what you need, and their perspectives are not critical here. Further, some friends and family members may have strong (and loud!) opinions and believe themselves experts on everything, including *you*. Be cautious, as their input can begin with (mis)understandings and viewpoints about the grief process, continue with ideas about what the next steps should—or shouldn't—be following your loss, and can include suggestions about the timing of your subsequent pregnancy.

TABITHA

After our daughter passed away, we were very withdrawn from family and society. The subsequent days and months were just us staying at home or doing things as a couple and not including others. Part of the reason for withdrawing

was that we did not feel others understood what we were going through, and
we did not want their unsolicited advice on how to grieve or continue on.

I felt like I was ready to go down the pregnancy road again not because I
wanted to replace the child I had, but because I wanted to become a parent to
a child I could actually raise. I did worry that people would judge me for trying
too soon after the loss of our daughter and I was fearful that if I went on to
have a healthy pregnancy and a healthy baby, people would forget about our
baby as well as everything we'd been through.

When talking with others about your plans to pursue another pregnancy, it is not unusual to feel judged, encouraged to wait, or even cautioned against trying again. Others may think that by allowing more time to pass, you will somehow have less grief and more strength to navigate another pregnancy. The unfortunate truth, as you well know, is that grief isn't always linear, it doesn't consistently decrease over time; on some level it is lifelong.

Following a tragedy that left third-degree burns over most of the body, it is understandable that bystanders would actively try to protect and dissuade the victim from even *looking* in the direction of fire. This can be especially prevalent in the case of recurrent pregnancy loss when some people cannot comprehend why in the world you would continue to place yourself in harm's way. They miss that you're also placing yourself in the way of *possibility* and it's because you want it so much that you are willing to tolerate the heat and the flames.

There are overt and covert messages offered that attempt to shield you, many of which are well-intended, but sting, upset, annoy, and offend you nonetheless:

"Maybe you should give this more time."
"You and your body have already been through so much."
"Have you thought about adoption?"
"Maybe it just wasn't meant to be?"
"I know you're still upset."

Of course, you are upset! You have just experienced the *loss of your pregnancy or death of your baby*! You know better than anyone that there are no guarantees in this life, not even with surrogacy or adoption. Moreover, you may understandably take offense at the suggestion that someone else's biological child (or another of your own) ever could or would become an even exchange for the one you just lost. Others are actually cautioning you against the idea of a "replacement baby" when they somehow suggest that you're considering trying too soon, but then send a mixed message when offering up adoption. The truth is that even if you had ten more children, none of them would ever replace or make up for the one you lost. There is no such thing as a replacement baby. There can be babies that follow, but every baby is unique and individual, and will forever hold his or her own place in your heart.

The people around you are all genuinely well intentioned, trying hard to be helpful, and protective of you and your best interests. But what they don't realize is if they encourage you to pursue anything other than another pregnancy, the loss multiplies as you then lose the opportunity to experience everything else related to that. For example, you'd lose the normal and natural experience of spontaneous conception, and/or the experience of pregnancy itself and the opportunity for a healthy delivery. You'd also lose the opportunity to parent for the first time (or to parent a sibling), and as important, the opportunity to regain a part of your identity and self-confidence that was deeply damaged by your loss.

Your sense of control, faith, and trust have all been shattered by your experience of loss. The system failed. Your body failed. You may even send yourself the message that you failed. By encouraging you or advising you to look away from the fire, you are temporarily afforded a reprieve from the daunting tasks of consideration of subsequent pregnancy and then the actual pursuit. These are things that at times may feel more complicated and complex than that of your grief. But it does you no favors in the long run, as your desire to have a child didn't die with the pregnancy or the lost baby. And this original desire and plan is something that may grow to haunt you if you don't find a way to confront and work through that fear, in spite of your grief.

It's okay to listen to others, but it's also okay to dismiss their advice. Ultimately, you must do what *you* feel to be best for *you*. Otherwise, you will only compound your grief, worry, fear, anxiety, and indecision with feelings of annoyance, frustration, bitterness, and then deep resentment. As miserable as it may feel right now, this is still *your* life. Talk as much and as often as you find helpful, but don't hesitate to pull back when you find others' input unhelpful. And finally, keep close to you those who listen well and consistently without judgment or unsolicited advice; their support will become more invaluable and treasured than ever.

MAKING THE RIGHT DECISION ABOUT TIMING FOR YOU

Once you are given the medical green light to begin trying again, you may still vacillate about when to start. As discussed in the previous chapter, there are many psychological and emotional considerations that are challenging to sort through. As you get closer to making a final decision about moving ahead, you may unexpectedly find yourself backtracking and questioning:

> *"Do I want this just because I don't have it?"*
> *"Do I want this because I'm trying to prove (to myself, or to others) that I can do it?"*
> *"Do I want this because I'm trying to escape my awful grief, or at least lessen it?"*
> *"Do I want this because changing the path of momentum feels too overwhelming, because if I'm not going to be a mother, well then what?"*

These types of questions generally stem from the increased fear you feel as you get closer to taking action, versus an indication of the need to change course. Although it's not impossible to change your mind, recognize that at this point, uncertainty is not only normal but also to be expected. Of course, you want to feel confident about taking such a big step and if you don't feel that way right now, questions will be inevitable.

Others' opinions and perspectives can create further personal uncertainty—you might immediately reject unhelpful comments, yet still struggle to forget them. You may not care what others think, but simultaneously be quite impressionable due to your increased vulnerability and decreased confidence.

You may also continue to worry about things that could go wrong. You have gained more knowledge and context since your loss. You've likely now been exposed to other women's stories of loss. Being a part of this unintended community of others with similar experiences can be incredibly helpful and supportive, particularly in you feeling less alone. However, this unique sisterhood can also compound your worry and fear because you are now aware of new and previously unknown risks and medical issues. More specifically, your list of things that can go wrong is multiplying. This can be overwhelming, even paralyzing. And it all makes for an awful lot of extra noise in your head.

It is critical to ensure you're moving forward not only for the right reason(s), but also toward the right destination. Individual therapy can help to more deeply explore your thoughts and feelings and affirm that the predominant reason(s) you want to proceed stem from a healthy foundation, such as a continuing desire for a baby/family.

Going through this decision process with your physician, your partner, and yourself plays a critical role in regaining a sense of confidence about yourself and your body, as well as your life. Other people's suggestions, even if well intentioned, have the potential to undermine your plans and rob you of your self-determination. This is challenging work, especially while you're feeling vulnerable, injured, and scared, but it's not impossible work.

So, aside from any medical recommendations that indicate concrete advantages of waiting, the decision to try again may simply be based on when you and your partner feel ready enough and willing to move forward once you've reaffirmed you do want a baby and a family. There will always be questions and fears, but at the end of the day, you will know you are ready when you can tell yourself that you want it more than you fear it.

AMY

The decision and process (even without infertility and loss) to start a family is such a challenge for a type A person like me. So, the thought of not knowing if and when a positive is going to come is such an emotional, nerve-racking experience. There is no control. As in NO CONTROL. Throw in recurrent pregnancy loss, and I'm truly shocked I have not gone insane. You're forced to just jump in because, at some point, there is no more thinking or planning or deciding, there is only doing.

There is no doubt you're feeling vulnerable, scared, and unsteady. As much as you don't want to be in this position, as you're learning, waiting can even magnify your anxieties by allowing them more time to grow. The truth is, it's going to be emotionally heart-wrenching no matter *when* you begin trying. There exists no "better" time; you are as ready as you will ever be to make these decisions, and it's time to start making them . . . now.

⸙ 4 ⸙

Getting Back (and Then Staying) in the Game

AT SOME POINT, EVERYONE HAS played a game . . . and then lost. There are different kinds of defeat, however. In some cases, people feel disappointment, but can find some comfort in the knowledge of a game they know and understand, and one they played well to the end. But there's another kind of defeat—just like what you experienced when you lost your pregnancy or baby. In this "game," the defeat was significantly worse not only because of what (who) you were playing for, but also because the rules were far from fair, and you weren't even allowed to play to the end. This is where the similarities to a game end, but the feelings of injustice remain deep and strong. The challenge here lies in finding a way back in, knowing you are going to keep at this until you win, all while hating everything about what it's going to take. What you also know is there's nothing simple or fun about this "game," especially when the stakes are so high and the outcome has the power to dramatically change the future of your life.

⸙ JESSICA

We are both heartbroken and devastated and left to ask the unfortunate questions of why and how this could happen again. We (and the doctors) believed the first time was a fluke and the chances of it happening again were like getting struck by lightning twice. Now we're left wondering if we will be able to have a healthy baby. This for me has been the most unbearable of all of it. I think after losing the first baby it was hard for us to accept that this was not just some terrible thing that happened to us that we had to get over, but something we were going to have to figure out how to live with.

There are two things I know for sure: we will try again, and I have no idea how we will ... but know that in time the answers will come. We will try again, we have to, I believe in it.

Hope and faith are curious notions that require belief and trust, two things that are often absent or inaccessible after the loss of a pregnancy or the death of a baby. You previously bought into and followed all the rules of engagement with your last pregnancy. Again, you played fair and gave it your all, and still, you didn't win. You were left empty-handed, feeling bitter and disillusioned. The quest for a subsequent pregnancy may now include the additional weight of anxiety, worry, fear, and feelings of desperation, obsession, and exhaustion. As scared and unsure as you may feel, you know you are going back in again ... but *how? How are you really going to do this?*

GETTING YOUR HEAD BACK IN THE GAME

The decision to begin trying again does not ensure that conception will occur. This is something every single woman knows that also creates a heightened state of vulnerability and fear. You may be spending considerable time and energy talking yourself (and others) back into this while simultaneously playing a mind game with yourself to ease your way back into uncertain territory. The two most common mind-sets at this time tend to be one of two extremes—forced positivity or self-protective pessimism.

Forced Positivity

You may somehow have gotten the idea into your head that conception is *only* going to occur if you wholeheartedly believe it will. You may consequently try to adopt unwavering positivity, working hard to extinguish every hint of anything other than a complete success. Although thoughts are indeed powerful, sheer mental will alone does not ensure conception. Possessing a positive mental attitude is great, but given your recent experience of loss, attempting to sustain a relentlessly positive demeanor may wind up creating even more pressure and stress.

QUINN

Everyone, including my husband, told me I needed to be positive when we were getting ready to try again. Everyone said if I continued to be negative and sad, I'd never conceive again, and if I did, it would be bad for the baby. Don't they know those things aren't helpful, and instead, haunt me? I'm already terrified of something bad happening again.

Self-Protective Pessimism

Alternatively, you may be cautious about allowing your expectations or hopes to grow too high and tell yourself and others, "*This is probably never going to work.*" You may further justify this stance by stating, "*I'm just being realistic.*" This is a deliberate attempt to avoid feeling too invested in or attached to the idea of something actually working for you so, in the event you don't conceive, the disappointment is mitigated. There is, however, no such thing as emotional preparedness if you don't conceive. Severe disappointment is inevitable, and you may then even blame yourself, believing it was somehow your fault for not having been more positive. Again, thoughts are powerful, but not that powerful.

You're wanting and focused on something that the overwhelming majority of the female species on this planet can achieve with ease and often without considerable effort. That is NOT an unreasonable want or expectation. If you don't conceive, the disappointment is not a result of your expectations somehow being too high, but rather, from the repeated fall from hope. While on some level these pessimistic beliefs may be heartfelt, they tend to be defense mechanisms. If there wasn't *any* hope, you would never try again and set yourself up for additional loss. The truth is that there *is* hope, but it can feel too big a risk, too great an exposure to acknowledge. This is part of the reason this pursuit is so challenging. By the sheer act of trying again, you are intentionally exposing yourself to risk and increased vulnerability.

JANE

I hate everything about this. I hate that I don't have my baby at home, and I hate that I have to start this fertility drill all over again. I damn the clinic as I sit here with all of my peers feeling angry yet trying to be hopeful, feeling exhausted but trying to stay determined, and still deeply sad. Everyone in the waiting area avoids eye contact. Everyone is sensitive to those who come back with strollers in tow, while the rest of us are still trying for our firsts, or for a baby we can keep at home because he/she actually lived. Everyone has a different story. And everyone's story is the same. I don't want to be this person who is dependent on medical technology to even have a shot at being a mother again, versus dependent on myself and my husband. I really don't think this is ever going to work. But at the end of the day, walking back into this clinic to do it all over again is the only thing imaginable that has the possibility of saving my life.

The best way to prepare yourself is to *be honest and real*. You have the power to consciously remove the pressure of having to think or feel a certain way. Recognize that your many mixed and complicated thoughts and feelings will continue to shift and change over time. Own that without judgment or analysis. Work to accept that reality, and *accept yourself* for where and who you are right now. Because of all you've lived through, it is normal and expected to experience a roller coaster of emotions for a very long time. It's both healthy and important for you to allow yourself a broader and more truthful range of expression about your full experience.

Remember, you've already made your decision to try again, and that momentum alone can carry you forward despite the noise that still exists in your head. If you're feeling scared and skeptical, acknowledge it, knowing you probably won't be able to outrun those reactions, and then work through them to the next step. In the event you can tap into a sense of hope, run with it as far as it will take you, but don't try to force yourself to always be positive. That can be exhausting. You'll be less stressed overall if you avoid forcing yourself to think or feel a certain way. Instead, work to preserve precious *and limited* reserves of energy rather than engage in mind games that can't and won't change the outcome.

HOW YOUR PAST EXPERIENCE CAN HELP

The past holds great significance for you as it will forever be associated with your lost pregnancy or deceased baby. But the past can also feel uncomfortable and unsafe because it contains feelings of failure and an experience of profound loss. The challenge here is to have your past be a part of you but not paralyze you. Revisiting the past—especially now—can help inform and shape your perspective in two important and useful ways as you move into action toward a subsequent pregnancy.

First, consider the example of operating a car and using the rearview mirror. Obviously, the best and safest practice is to primarily focus on the road ahead while looking through the front windshield. But there are reasons why cars are also equipped with rearview mirrors—they are crucial in navigation and designed to enhance a car's safety, as long as the driver uses them to maintain perspective on the road. By looking at your recent experience with a rearview frame of reference, you (and your physician) can better assess if there is—or isn't—anything that can be done differently in a subsequent pregnancy, and if there is, to act on it.

Second, your past experiences will help reinforce a more accurate and complete perspective of yourself. Looking through the rear mirror at this point will confirm that *some* time has passed since your loss, whether that is days, weeks, months, or a year or two. As surreal as time feels, *you are surviving the worst thing ever.* You may feel beaten down, but you are still breathing. You are getting through your days even though they are hard, painful, and seemingly impossible at times. You don't see your resilience or endurance, but those traits *are* somewhere inside you, and you have been using them (even if unconsciously) to get through each day from your loss to today. Even if buried by the weight of your grief, those strengths are still in there, actively working on their own, and they will be useful in navigating the journey ahead (and eventually in rebuilding self-esteem and confidence) without you having to do anything just yet.

One note of caution: As you prepare to take active steps forward, it's wise to be careful when using your mirror. There is a reason the front view is of greater scope and size than the rear-facing mirror, and these views must be kept in proper balance. You may need to be reminded of this fact and encouraged to shift your sights forward accordingly as you prepare to actively begin trying for another pregnancy. This in no way suggests lessening the importance of the past, but instead helps remind you of the safest way to face as you prepare to put the car back into drive.

BUILDING (OR REBUILDING) YOUR RELATIONSHIP WITH YOUR PHYSICIAN

No one likes a backseat driver but sometimes having another person in the car can be helpful. This is especially true when it comes to your relationship with your physician. Whether you are starting with someone new, or rebuilding and strengthening your relationship with your original physician, this person is going to be critical throughout your next pregnancy. You've already completed the work to identify who you are going to work with, and now is the time to actively lean into this relationship. Regardless of any hesitancy you may have to trust anything (or anyone) in the medical system, your physician is going to be one of the two people closest to you through this next pregnancy, and ultimately, a deepened relationship with him or her will help you feel less alone. Starting all over again is tough, especially when you are acutely aware of all the things you can't control. Do your best to focus on the following things you *can* control and then actively do, including:

1. **Schedule a "preconception consultation" with your physician.** This appointment should be scheduled now as you will be less distracted and anxious than after conception. At this visit, a physician will often check

immunization titers, blood type, and consider genetic carrier panels. This is also a good opportunity to discuss risk factors in pregnancy and optimize any underlying medical conditions. You should discuss your plan to begin attempts for conception (identifying any needed medical assistance), and also request that your physician clearly outline his/her plan for the medical management of this next pregnancy. In addition, use this time to address your anticipated emotional needs (for example, more frequent appointments at sensitive gestational milestones). Clarifying how and what you're feeling, along with expressing what is and isn't helpful, will assist your physician and his or her staff in providing better and more personalized care now and throughout the subsequent pregnancy. This candid conversation will help ensure you are both on the same page moving forward. Should you discover you're not, you will have a broad window of time in which to continue talking and working toward a mutually agreeable resolution. Even though you won't be able to control everything on the road ahead, discussing a plan for navigating some of the potential sharp curves will make a big difference emotionally as you pace yourself through another pregnancy. Finally, if desired, this appointment may also include a review and discussion of your last pregnancy and loss if you have not already had this conversation, or if you deem it helpful.

2. **Create opportunities, now and throughout your pregnancy, to ask your physician whatever questions you have.** Provide your physician with a copy of your questions at the beginning of your appointments and ask, *"Will you please help me manage our time today? I have a lot of questions."* Do not cheat yourself by pretending you don't have a long list of questions. Present ALL of your questions and gauge your physician's response and demeanor. If your physician is rushed at the preconception consultation and seems annoyed by the length of your list, he/she is likely not right for you. If this is the case, it's better to learn this sooner than later. Your physician can quickly review your list at the beginning of your appointments and help organize the questions—and the conversation—to address your concerns and then help you focus on

what is most relevant for you medically. Push yourself to be honest and transparent, even if full disclosure makes you feel somewhat needy. The goal of the preconception consultation is to clarify the medical plan going forward and also confirm your choice in physicians. It is normal to have doubts and concerns given all you've been through, but it's critical to explore whether or not you trust this person enough to place yourself under his/her care. If not, take the time necessary to find another physician.

3. **Clarify expectations regarding future communication and contact with your physician.** Having your physician's office phone number may mean different things. Some physicians have patients primarily communicate with their nurses, assistants, or front desk staff. Many physicians communicate directly through a secure online portal or will return calls after office hours. Confirm your understanding of the office protocol for communication and the time frame for response. If it's vital for you to speak with your physician directly at times, determine the preferred way to do so to avoid potential confusion, disappointment, or angst in the future.

STRENGTHENING YOUR RELATIONSHIP WITH YOUR PARTNER

Maintaining open and proactive lines of communication with your partner is critical to your relationship, but this does not mean you have to talk about your efforts for pregnancy all the time and every single day. Find a cadence for communication that works for you both, knowing it may be helpful to take time off from talking about or focusing on pregnancy. Find ways to connect and be together that aren't layered under the weight of trying, like watching movies, cooking, or taking walks. As you work to establish a healthy balance, just remember to:

1. **Check in with yourself and your partner between attempts at conception, to reaffirm or revise the game plan, if needed.** Your thoughts and feelings (and those of your partner) may continue to change unexpectedly. Your decision to try again and discussions with your physician should not lock you into an unalterable plan of action

if you or your partner suddenly discover you want or need a temporary break. There is enough pressure in this process already without creating more of your own. A brief pause or a rest cycle is not unreasonable. Communicate openly with your partner to identify the next window of ovulation or open IVF cycle if the current one feels like too much for either of you.

ALLY

I'm a realistic person. I knew we wouldn't get pregnant on our first cycle once we returned to IVF. What I didn't know was, as the months passed, I would find things even bigger than my grief: I found even more anxiety and depression. Trying and trying and trying again had pushed me into a vicious cycle of either trying to get pregnant or being disappointed. My husband said we just have to keep going. I said I can't keep doing this, I need a break.

That month off was awful. My husband was angry but quiet, even though he denied it. I thought he hated me; I hated myself, and I knew we both hated our situation. Somehow, we got through it though.

When I got my period the next month, I cried and cried and then blamed myself for the lost opportunity telling myself that that was the month we would have gotten pregnant. I was surprised, but my husband sat and held me while I cried. He said he wasn't angry at me. He was angry we had lost our daughter, and he felt bad and sad for us all. He was angry that we had to go through this all again, and wanted to protect me from that, but was angry he couldn't. He also said he was angry with himself for not sharing any of this before.

I don't know if we would have talked about these things if we hadn't taken that cycle off. We might instead have just kept everything locked inside and used the little energy we had for trying. As hard as that month was, I think in the end, it was also helpful.

2. **Recognize and proactively discuss realistic expectations for intimacy during this time of active attempts.** This will work to minimize the potential for assumptions and miscommunications. Trying again

won't likely be relaxing or enjoyable, especially if you are going through fertility treatment, but that does not signal the end of a healthy sex life—you can and will get that back in time. It just means *now* may not be that time. This period can be stressful and loaded with pressure for you both. It may be dominated by frustrations and fears given what you have been through. Be as patient and supportive of each other as you can be. Express the things most helpful for you (for example, skipping the foreplay and instead focusing your limited energies on ejaculation). Also ask your partner what he/she needs from you and then try to provide that to the greatest extent possible. Continue to remind yourselves that you are on the same team and actively working toward the same end goals, which include not only another pregnancy but also a strong and solid partnership.

ERIN

We were pretty aggressive, from a medical standpoint, once we decided to try again. I felt behind where I wanted to be with having children and knew that it wasn't going to get any easier to conceive the older I got. If I waited until I was emotionally ready (whatever that means), I could miss my chance to have another child. And we didn't want our living children to be too far apart in age. Also, I hadn't gotten my period again since our daughter was born five months prior and I wanted to know now if something was wrong. My OB said not to worry, it was probably just stress, and to give myself time to ovulate again. That was not acceptable for me. Stress was part of my life, and that wasn't going away anytime soon. I needed to take some control of the situation, and I knew my OB wouldn't be as aggressive as I wanted, so we went to a reproductive endocrinologist for all the appropriate testing and worked directly with them to get pregnant. Trying to get pregnant again was not enjoyable and I wanted to minimize that part of the process as best we could. The idea of getting pregnant with a child that we wouldn't be having had our daughter lived took any of the enjoyment out of the process and replaced it with guilt and a whole lot of anger and anxiety.

TAKING CARE OF AND MONITORING YOUR BODY

Continue to take good care of yourself. That includes what you do with your body and what you put into it. Remain active and exercise regularly because a healthy body will provide you a stronger base from which to handle emotional challenges. Get plenty of rest so that you have enough energy to get through each day. Stay well hydrated and nourish yourself with healthy and nutritious foods. Be aware that controlled eating can become extreme, especially if you are using it to compensate for feeling a lack of control in many other areas of your life right now. The overall focus should be on healthy eating and living but remind yourself that perfection is not realistic.

LIA

I'm struggling with all of these daily decisions. What should I eat and what should I drink? Is having a coffee okay or not? How much exercise is good? How much is too much? I'm driving myself crazy overthinking and then second-guessing every single choice I make. But I will never forgive myself if there is another bad outcome and there was something I could have done differently because then I'll blame myself.

It is good for you to be knowledgeable about your body and to self-monitor to determine the best window for ovulation, assuming this does not create more stress for you. Home ovulation predictor kits work well for some women but significantly increase anxiety for others. In the event you are experiencing anxiety over identifying your ovulation window, consider asking your physician for a midcycle scan to assess for follicle growth, and then obtain a recommendation for optimally timed intercourse as this can remove some of the guesswork and provide you with some relief.

Review the plan you mapped out with your physician (such as, trying for spontaneous conception for six months), and revisit that if or as needed. Six months of trying on your own may start to feel like six years, so if you find yourself wanting to call your physician's office after four months of unsuccessful attempts, don't hesitate to initiate this contact. It is understandable to want to explore other—and potentially more aggressive—options if the current plan isn't working.

Finally, recognize that most women have little patience at this point, and will be susceptible to stress-related anxiety and compulsive internet searches that only exacerbate worries. It is best to avoid self-diagnosis. If you don't conceive as straightforwardly as you wish, your mind will likely go to the worst-case scenario, entertaining catastrophic thoughts such as *"Now I'm going to have to deal with infertility too!"* Even though you know your body well at this point, you are still the patient, not the physician. A series of unsuccessful attempts for conception is just that—it does not necessarily mean you are going to have to deal with infertility on top of loss. Again, talk with your physician and set aside any information that is not relevant for you.

ᘒ IF YOU HAVE STRUGGLED WITH INFERTILITY ᘒ

You've already been shouldering worst-case scenario thoughts for some time. Although you don't have a guarantee that you're going to conceive again, you do have something that many women struggling with infertility don't yet have. You have the knowledge and the experience that you *can*, and *did*, conceive. It's normal and natural for you to focus on the infertility and loss part of your history, fixating on your worry that you won't ever be able to conceive again. Your history, however, includes a good reminder and evidence that you can.

STAYING IN THE GAME EMOTIONALLY

For most women, delays in conception are upsetting and discouraging—even more so after being given the medical clearance to begin trying again and then being unsuccessful month after month. Self-confidence can erode rapidly and anxieties race ever higher. Hitting wall after wall, but knowing the only way to succeed is to keep trying, pushes you to keep investing your efforts and your time. It is an incredibly defeating and numbing sensation to watch your emotional savings diminish while actively participating in that process. Emotional resilience, stamina, and endurance become critical at this time. But how can you access and then enhance those things when you are already feeling emotionally exhausted and depleted?

Get a Good Therapist

If you haven't already, find someone who is knowledgeable and experienced in the area of women's mental and reproductive health, and schedule regular appointments. Although a therapist can't change the path, she or he can prove invaluable as you remain on it, offering you support and guidance through the inevitable sharp curves and difficult stretches ahead. (If you find yourself overwhelmed with symptoms of anxiety and/or depression, you might also consider consulting with a licensed and board-certified psychiatrist who has expertise in medical and obstetric care to explore and prescribe medication.)

Practice Proper Self-Care Regularly

Most women are raised and socialized to put others' needs and wants before their own. This is an altruistic trait that can be a double-edged sword. Instead of focusing outward, you're going to need to shift that focus inward and *put yourself first*. This is critical to your mental/physical health and survival. Chances are, you may feel that you are running on fumes after losing a pregnancy or following the death of your baby, and those fumes should not be used up on others' wants. Instead, they should be focused on *your needs* and *your wants*. It's not only about putting yourself first; it's also about taking good care of yourself in many ways, whether it's sleeping more, eating better, scheduling a spa day, heading to that yoga class, or treating yourself to something special. Grab whatever fleeting moments you can to be good to yourself as that will help you better handle what is ahead. If you're going to reenter and then finish this race and finish strong, you will need all the fuel you can get. Self-care should be practiced regularly and frequently. Being patient, gentle, and kind, but also generous with yourself should become standard and daily, not just on special occasions, such as birthdays or anniversaries.

⸓ A NOTE ON STRESS MANAGEMENT ⸓

After a loss, you are keenly aware of your stress levels, and your inability to effectively control them. You're also mindful of the potential negative impact of stress on yourself regarding conception and any future pregnancy. Although it is best for you to have the lowest stress levels possible, efforts to conceive will be riddled with anxiety and uncertainty. Once you've experienced trauma and loss, future possible negative outcomes may now feel probable. Ideally, your time should be spent working with your therapist and finding ways to better manage and tolerate the high stress, versus the unrealistic goal of low stress. The truth is that people all around the world do conceive during times of extraordinary anxiety and extreme stress and still go on to deliver healthy babies.

Improve Self-Awareness

It is vital to regularly reflect on how and what you are feeling and to assess your honest reactions to the world around you, including people and situations. You may not always know what is helpful, but you can at least identify some of the things that *aren't* (such as seeing a pregnant friend or attending a large social event), and then allow yourself more distance. Keep in mind that your feelings toward things, people, and situations may change unexpectedly. You may continue to feel hypersensitive, and one comment or unintended word choice may cause you to step back or disengage entirely. It may be confusing, unexpected, and uncomfortable for you (and those around you) to recognize some of the things that aren't helpful at times, including interactions with your best friend. However, that knowledge can help you avoid setting yourself up for repeated disappointment and discomfort. Remember, you are the one who is hurting, and you should not feel obliged to compromise your emotional health to please anyone. That will only result in more hurt and eventual resentment. Awareness of your triggers is the first step in helping you temporarily sidestep things, people, and situations that cause you more discomfort or even pain at this time.

ALLISON

Although I never truly suffered from infertility, when we began to try to get pregnant again, there were four periods that came and went, that signified I wasn't pregnant yet. Each time I utterly lost control—I had angry outbursts and became erratic with friends and coworkers. In many ways, it was the time where my emotions flowed as they couldn't during the limited days between our prenatal diagnosis and D&E. Each day seemed to be mixed with fear, hope, and obsession. I could not tolerate being around babies or children, I could not attend baby showers. (This reaction was so intense that even now—after having two baby showers and three children of my own—I feel a loss of control of my emotions when birth announcements or baby showers occur.)

Self-Advocate

As you clarify and confirm the things, people, and situations that are not helpful, do not be afraid to stand up, speak up, step back, or temporarily step away. You do not owe others a reason, an explanation, or a justification. But if you feel you must say something, sample language might include:

> *"I'm sorry to interrupt you; I need to take a break/use the bathroom/get some water, fresh air, etc."*
> *"I'm having trouble concentrating right now; I'll be back in touch when I can."*
> *"It's difficult to RSVP right now as I can't anticipate how I'm going to be feeling. If you need a final head count today, then my answer will have to be no."*
> *"I received your invite but unfortunately, I won't be able to attend. I'm sure your party will be lovely; you're always such a generous host."*
> *"Excuse me, I need to get off the phone now. All of a sudden, I'm just exhausted." or "It's time for me to head home."*

You owe it to yourself to buffer and shield your already vulnerable head, heart, and body. Expending time and energy on others without benefit to yourself will further deplete and drain your limited reserves, and increase feelings of anger. Self-advocacy is all about knowing yourself, your needs, and your wants, and then allowing yourself to get them met. Anticipate that others may not fully accept your responses and may try to persuade you to do things that are not comfortable for you. Remember, *you* are the only one who knows what it feels like to put on your shoes each day; no one else has had to wear them. Maybe someone walked next to you for part of the way or had shoes that looked similar, but they're not *yours*. Only *you* know what your needs and wants are, and it's important to recognize they are as important as anyone else's. When you're bereaved, you have limited energy and may be unable to tap into and replenish your reserves regularly. Therefore, during this time, it is critical to be highly selective and discretionary about what you agree to do and with whom. You can be kind, but direct. Thoughtful, but assertive. Loving, but centered on the things most helpful for *you*. Empower yourself to put your needs first. There is *no one* more important than you right now.

Strive for Balanced Identity

As you continue efforts for self-advocacy, remind yourself that you have other parts to your identity—besides fertility—that you should advocate for as well. Ideally, the act of trying again should be a *part* of your life, rather than *becoming* your life. This is an extraordinary challenge when you've lost not just a pregnancy or a baby, but all other parts of yourself, including your interests, activities, and your mojo in general. It's vital to find some balance, even if you define yourself by motherhood. If the worst-case scenario occurs—that you don't conceive—then you have other parts of your identity on which to lean and eventually build. But if you have no other interests/ activities, the time invested in the conception process can seem in vain and make you feel even emptier and further defeated. The best-case scenario: successfully find interests and activities that will help fill your time through your efforts to conceive and the nine months of pregnancy to follow. Staying busy and productive encourages your return to the multidimensional woman you truly are. Once a week, strive to carve out at least one to two hours to focus on an activity that is new and has nothing to do with pregnancy. For example, shop for ingredients and prepare a brand-new recipe you haven't yet made, or go to the library and find a good book that may temporarily distract you as you immerse yourself in a world or story far removed from your own. Admittedly, you may have no interest or energy for anything outside the pursuit of another pregnancy, but placing yourself in situations where a spark may be ignited is a start.

EVERYONE HAS CHALLENGES

Chances are, many people around you didn't know what to say or do after your loss. This is evidenced by a common statement that inadvertently put all the responsibility on you: *"Please let me know if there's anything you need."* While sincere and well intended, this comment assumes you would know what your needs are or be able to ask for help when you're in free fall. You may feel frustrated to be in a position of having to educate others, but others can't read your mind to know what is most useful (or unhelpful) at any given time.

As you attempt another pregnancy, others close to you will sincerely want to be helpful and supportive, and encourage you in ways *they* believe to be helpful and supportive:

"Don't worry—you'll be able to have another baby."
"You just have to relax and it will happen."
"I know this next pregnancy/baby will be healthy."
"Well, if it doesn't work, there's always adoption."

Once-trusted networks of support—even your own mother—may unexpectedly and repeatedly disappoint by saying the wrong thing. Even when you have the energy to give specific direction, others may fumble. In their defense, they are doing their absolute best. They sincerely want you to get better, to feel better, and to find happiness. But you may experience these types of comments and messages of intended comfort as placating, grating, and offensive. Despite the good intentions, no one can ensure a successful outcome.

Your strong reactions to others will not likely be limited to their comments on you trying again, or another pregnancy. It may be *especially* difficult for you to tolerate news about others' pregnancies, in addition to finding you have little bandwidth to hear about *anything* going on in anyone else's life right now. This includes news of an engagement, a wedding, or a death in someone else's family. You may realize you have exactly *nothing* to add to the conversation or give to the person when you're feeling so emotionally fragile and empty. This lack of empathy is not uncommon following loss or trauma, but it can result in you carrying more guilt, even feelings of shame.

Your unexpected hurt or anger, or atypical disengagement, may arouse frustration and confusion in others. They may feel they are unable to do anything right or well in the face of your unanticipated, unpredictable, and misunderstood reactions to their well-intended desire to reach out to you, engage you, and include you. Those who love you most want you to remain an active and involved part of their lives, and they in yours. So, they're going to continue to try to communicate with you even if, at times, you find it impossible to respond, engage, or participate.

Because of this push-pull dynamic, you may find yourself distancing and isolating yourself from your own support network to avoid the unintended hurts others may continue to inflict. And yet, hiding out from the rest of the world is not a realistic or healthy option long term. *So, what's your role here? Do you still have any responsibility to others, and if so, what?*

JENNY

I remember feeling like EVERYONE around me was pregnant after my loss, had the same/similar due date as mine—social life was painful, work life was painful, every encounter felt awkward and strained and fake. I found comfort in friends/people who were going through something "abnormal" too. It's been weird what feels good and what doesn't and who I feel like seeing and who I don't . . . I feel like I'm being selfish and a bad friend/worker. I'm starting to feel like I need to "snap out" of my sadness, but I keep having all these feelings that

I don't recognize/feel comfortable with. I talked to my [pregnant] girlfriend last week, which was hard. The actual conversation was good but I feel more alienated now that I've said everything I wanted to say; that it hurt my feelings that I found out she was having a boy on Facebook and that I really didn't feel up to all these group things she was planning but that I'd like to hang out one-on-one. I haven't heard from her since but I think she doesn't really know what to do or say. I also emailed my husband's pregnant sister to apologize for being a bad sister-in-law in sharing their exciting news. Her pregnancy is like the elephant in the room, and I feel bad and high maintenance that everyone is avoiding it (even though I don't feel strong enough to talk about it). I feel so selfish—like all these people are having to tip-toe around me, and I don't know how to feel or just be normal.

STRATEGIES FOR RESPONSE AND ENGAGEMENT

At a time you could benefit from support more than ever, your reality may be that nothing and no one feels safe because you are so easily triggered and hypersensitive to feeling alone in a place you didn't choose or want—all while you witness others continuing to advance in their own lives ahead of you. Although unconditional and unchallenged support is important, and valued by you now more than ever, not everyone will be able to always extend that to you. You're going to have to make some decisions about whether or not you respond, engage in, or even continue various relationships, and if so, how to go about doing it.

Who to Prioritize

First and foremost, your responsibility is to yourself and your partner. Period. Yet, both of you will need additional support through this process if you're going to make it through intact. And even though others may have hurt you, you *do* have meaningful people in your life who you ultimately will want to keep. You *will* lose relationships if you exclusively adopt the attitude of *"I'll show up when I want, and when I do you have to give me exactly what I need and want, otherwise I'm not coming back.*" Always be mindful and selective about the people and situations you prioritize, using your energy for those most important to you. To do this, begin working from the inside out.

Draw an imaginary line that forms a circle around yourself and your partner, and any other children you have. Then, consider the depth, duration, integrity, and status of all other active relationships you have. Create a series of concentric rings drawn outward, moving from most intimate to least intimate, and determine where to place each of these people, if at all.

During this process, you may discover that some relationships require more effort than they're worth, so this is an excellent time to take inventory and release yourself from connections that give you little, if anything, in return. The process can be an eye-opener because, until now, you may have unconsciously been more tolerant and less focused on the actual merits of the relationship to have ever considered stepping back or out. Some of your choices may now surprise you—a longtime but somewhat distant friend of many years may not make the cut, whereas a newer but very thoughtful friend may prove worthy of drawing in closer. As you have the time and energy, keep this process going until you have a clear sense of those who are worth your time and attention.

⟨ WHERE DOES FAMILY FIT? ⟩

Sometimes, your relationships with your family members are the most triggering. If that is the case, give the minimum required of your presence or participation, and ensure you have buffers (such as an accompanying partner) when you do engage. Unless the relationship is abusive or toxic, family is still family, and fracturing the relationship with your mother-in-law because of her insensitivities will only create more tension in your relationship with your partner. As hard as it can be, keep in mind that you don't get to choose your family members, and the reality is they're going to be around for a while.

What to Prioritize

No exact formula exists that will help you determine where your priorities should lie, but here are the two most important situations to consider:

1. Major life events and milestones of people closest to you
2. Situations where your absence would draw even more (negative) attention to you

For example, your presence at your grandmother's funeral is a priority; your presence at your annual office party is optional. Acknowledging a cousin's or friend's pregnancy is the right thing to do, even if done via text or email; your presence at the baby shower might warrant a decline. Use common sense and discretion.

But what happens if that baby shower is for your sister or best friend of twenty years? As hard as it may feel in this case, "doing the right thing" and attending may ultimately create less stress for you, than fielding others' unending questions before and after the event. If you don't think you can hold it together for a few hours, bow out gracefully in advance rather than force yourself to go through the motions only to create a scene later. Talk with your partner to reconcile your perspectives, and talk to your therapist who can help you explore these decisions from a more objective standpoint.

When to Prioritize

You always have the option to ignore a comment or situation or to respond and engage. However, if you decide to acknowledge a seemingly helpful comment or gesture, you increase the chance for more because the sender will feel his/her efforts have been validated.

If you identify an unhelpful comment or contact, before responding (or deciding not to), clarify your intentions and your expectation of others. More specifically, if you feel your response should result in the other person somehow apologizing for or changing their words, actions, or behaviors, you may be setting yourself up for further disappointment unless you believe, wholeheartedly, they would be so receptive.

A more realistic goal may be to share information about your experience because this is something you can control. You may hope for increased sensitivity and a change in interactions, but understand that's not guaranteed. Thoughtful and selective disclosures do not always produce desired results, but are merely a way for you to take back some control and potentially gain more support during this journey.

How to Politely but Directly Respond When Triggered

There are endless examples of people's good intentions that may leave you feeling upset and uncomfortable. Here are some of the more common ones and suggested responses, if you are confronted with them:

"Don't worry—you'll be able to have another baby."
Suggested response: *"My worry is going to be around for a long time and is not something I can turn off right now. I know your words are meant to be encouraging when you tell me you know I'm going to have another baby. It's tough for me to keep hearing that because the reality is no one knows that for sure. It's actually more helpful to hear that you love me and that you're here for me."*

"You just have to relax and it will happen."
Suggested response: *"Even if I was able to feel relaxed for a time, my reality is the stress is going to continue and will increase after conception. That is a lingering part of the trauma I have experienced. I can't ask you to understand that, I'm just asking that you try."*

"I know this next pregnancy/baby will be healthy."
Suggested response: *"I wish I had that kind of a guarantee but no one can provide me with one. I'm focused on taking care of myself right now. Having you recognize and acknowledge how hard I'm working to keep myself healthy is actually more encouraging for me."*

"My friend's daughter had a miscarriage and now she's pregnant again."

Suggested response: *"I'm sorry for her loss, but her situation has nothing to do with mine. Sharing that only reminds me that bad things happen. I'm already focused on my own medical situation, so it's not helpful to keep hearing about others'. It's more helpful to have you ask and then listen to how I'm doing."*

"Well, if it doesn't work, there's always adoption."

Suggested response: *"I know you're trying to be encouraging but that's not our focus. We are trying to have a biological child. Further, the truth is there are no guarantees with adoption, either. It's more helpful for me to hear that others understand and are behind the choices we've made for ourselves."*

"I want to share the good news with you—I'm pregnant."

Suggested response: *"I'm hopeful for everything ahead of you. However, pregnancy remains a very sensitive area for me, and I need to step back temporarily. Please don't take that personally. I hope our friendship can weather the short-term distance, but I'm not able to be the friend I'd ideally want to be right now."*

"Please think about coming to my baby shower. It would mean so much to me if you were there."

Suggested response: *"I'm sorry, but no. I care enough about you to be honest. Please understand, this is nothing against you; it's just too painful for me. I'm not willing to take any focus away from you and don't trust my emotions given where I'm at right now."*

"I really want to see you. When can we get together?"

Suggested response: *"Thank you for thinking of me. I have to be honest—I'm just not up for it right now, but will let you know when I'm ready."*

Or *"It's really difficult for me to predict in advance how I'm going to be feeling on any given day. Would you be willing to set a date and time, but confirm the day of, in case I need to reschedule?"*

It can be awkward and uncomfortable to be so direct with others, but if you assess the relationship first and deem it strong enough to tolerate such honesty, you might find some relief and release. Even if the person doesn't perfectly hear your message, you are practicing increased assertion and interpersonal effectiveness, which will continue to help you along this path. You now have the capacity to be candid when you feel you must. Remember, harbored resentments are like springs; the more they are pushed down, the greater the tension and the stronger the force. Adding resentment and anger to your grief is not going to serve you; it's simply more weight for you to carry.

A FINAL MESSAGE TO YOU AND ALL THE OTHERS WHO SURROUND YOU: PERSEVERE

It's not always going to feel or be like this. Courageous resolution—steeling yourself for the long haul—is an important concept for you and those closest to you to embrace. You know with every fiber of your being you are going to keep trying until you conceive. This has never been in question. Instead, the real issue is how you're going to emotionally pace yourself and navigate the relationships and the world around you during attempts to conceive. You will find your footing and your longer-term path if you're honest with yourself and identify the things, people, and situations that are and are not helpful. Be selective and use your limited reserves wisely. Focus on yourself first and then prioritize the needs of others closest to you when you are able to give something back to them. Releasing yourself from relationships that don't feel reciprocal or balanced will free up some energy that you can use toward those relationships that matter most.

Your patience may have been exhausted a long time ago, but your persistence has not. Although you have little control over time frames and final outcomes, there are some things you *can* control. You can remind yourself that not conceiving now does not mean not ever. You can recognize that by deciding to try again and then beginning attempts, you are taking action—regardless of whether you feel optimistic, or nervous and doubtful. You can continue to put one foot in front of the other, just as you've done every single day since your loss, even though you feel defeated and exhausted. You can find ways to run with your pursuit of pregnancy and not have the pursuit run you. Trying to conceive again (and perhaps again and again) can feel like the beginning of the most insane endurance sport ever. Staying the course doesn't guarantee a win, but it *does* guarantee you still have a *chance*.

⸎ 5 ⸎

The Results Are In: Pregnancy Testing and Its Aftermath

STURM UND DRANG IS A German phrase that means "storm and stress" or, more simply, "turmoil." This term exactly describes the experience of pregnancy testing as either negative or positive pregnancy results can trigger equally intense and stressful feelings. No matter the outcome, you are faced with a challenge—whether navigating the growing disappointment of having to try again next month, or beginning the nerve-racking roller-coaster ride of pregnancy ahead. Either scenario puts extraordinary pressure on this "yes or no" moment.

⸎ THE WAIT TO TEST ⸎

Few admit this, but many women take a home pregnancy test *before* the earliest recommended date, or before their scheduled blood test at their physician's office if undergoing fertility treatments. This is because the wait can feel too long to bear. Be aware, however, that early results are not always accurate or reliable, and if you receive a false positive or a false negative, you may wind

(continues)

(continued)

up unintentionally increasing your depression and anxiety. Some medications (including certain ones used during fertility treatments) may remain in your system and can influence your results if you test too early. Do your best to hang on until the recommended date. Even if you end up without the result you wanted, that's ultimately going to be less to manage than adding the tormenting tease or subsequent whiplash of a false reading.

Every woman opens the home pregnancy test box or awaits the blood test result with great trepidation and a deep well of varied emotions because she knows there is going to be a powerful reaction, whatever the outcome. The already charged news of a positive or negative result will land on existing strong emotion, and an awful lot of context carried over from your previous loss will serve to further intensify both experiences. No matter how much time has passed, you're still carrying your loss experience. Even though you want a positive result more than anything, you might not realize the depth of your lingering vulnerability until it becomes a fact, staring you hard in the face, and leaving you to figure out how to deal with it.

LIV

I refer to that year as the year of loss. It was one fucking bad year. First, my baby daughter died. Then my mom died after a long battle with cancer. Then, my beloved geriatric dog died. Two were devastating but expected. One still makes absolutely no fucking sense, and on some level, I don't think I will ever recover.

Everyone kept telling me, "Bad things happen in threes." So, I told myself once we started trying again that I HAD to get pregnant. It just HAD to happen. I mean, come on. What more could I deal with?

As fate would have it, I then had to deal with a negative pregnancy test result SIX MONTHS IN A ROW. Turns out bad things don't always happen in threes. For me, it seemed they happened in multiples of three.

The potential layers of disappointment and heartache run deep, and a negative test only adds to the growing list of loss. Active and continuing grief frequently overlaps and, at times, can even overshadow subsequent attempts at conception. Many women hope and believe that conception will mark a time of new beginning and help reduce their grief. However, on some level, the grief continues, and reactions can intensify around the time of pregnancy testing as the past, present, and future intersect. There is also the added weight of processing the actual test result and then having to take the next steps once a clear direction is determined.

⸂ YOUR DUE DATES ⸃

Every woman is aware of her prior due date and the projected due date of this pregnancy (if conception occurs), and the relationship between them. Some women intentionally avoid trying before their prior due date, out of respect for their deceased baby or due to feelings of guilt. Other women feel an increased sense of urgency to be pregnant in advance of this day, believing the pain of their grief will somehow be more bearable and that they'll find some small comfort in having taken action to get back on course.

If your pregnancy test result is negative, you may feel not only disappointment, but also the increasing anxiety of advancing ever closer to the edge of a reproductive window. This only adds more pressure and emotional charge to the results. This is especially true for women who intentionally avoid conception before their original due date. Most still end up disappointed when that due date nears as they are acutely aware of the passage of time and the fact that they still have nothing to show for it, despite all their efforts to date.

FACING THE RESULTS
Negative News

A negative pregnancy test result can deepen depression and exacerbate anxiety and feelings of hopelessness. The sickening but familiar sensation of despair can also be confusing. You believed you had already hit rock bottom following your loss, but the cumulative pull from your current (or recurrent) setback can plunge you even deeper. Negative results can damage your ego and overall sense of identity. *"I didn't know it was possible to feel even worse about myself, and about my life."*

After feeling discouraged, defeated, and hopeless, you may find yourself struggling to act during a subsequent window of ovulation, only to later blame yourself and feel deep regret for missing that window. You may compensate by forcing yourself to try again, with even greater commitment and vigilance the following month. Or you may consider a temporary break.

If you have experienced the repeated disappointment of negative results, you may benefit from additional support and counseling during this time to help process your reactions and develop strategies to better regulate your emotions and improve your ability to tolerate stress and uncertainty. Further, therapy can be useful in exploring the pros and cons of a short break. Taking some time off doesn't mean taking steps backward or taking yourself out of the conception race; instead, it's about focusing on what is needed to keep you in the race.

In addition to adverse reactions to a negative test, you may experience something entirely unanticipated—a sensation of actual *relief*. When trying again, high levels of anticipatory anxiety can exist, and these anxieties only heighten once another pregnancy is confirmed. Following a negative test, and despite desperately wanting another pregnancy, you may feel relieved that you don't have to face nine months of increasing anxiety. This reaction may even make you question yourself: *"If this is how I feel, does it mean I really don't want another baby?"*

This feeling of relief usually has more to do with a temporary lifting of distress (caused by the weight of navigating another pregnancy) than your emotions about conceiving again. Because, if you're really being honest with yourself, you know you're going to continue trying until you are pregnant. In the event you find your emotions starting to stray off course, pay attention to them and confirm you have the determination and resilience to forge forward instead of just throwing yourself back into another attempt.

The Decision to Change Course

Every woman who has experienced loss knows she has no guarantee she will conceive again or even have another baby. This is a harsh reality, but one you already recognize. Again, after a loss, most women will resume attempts to conceive. But for how long? Especially if there are more setbacks?

Every woman has a unique upper limit, and you're not going to know yours until you reach it. Many variables can impact this decision, including your health and medical status, as well as finances. Some women say, *"I'll give this one more try, and if it doesn't work, I'm done."* That's fine, but it's also fine to wait and see where you're at after that try as you may find more will or another way to continue.

Depending on your circumstances, your path toward this next baby may include challenges with repeat conception, or you may be advised your best chances involve the use of donor egg, sperm, or embryos, surrogacy, or the use of a gestational carrier. Your path may include the pursuit of private adoption. Instead of viewing these options on some continuum from best to worst, see them as different pathways toward the same meaningful end goal: creation of your family.

It's also possible your path may even include one or more repeat losses before bringing home a healthy full-term baby. There might be another biological loss, one experienced through a surrogate or gestational carrier, or even while pursuing adoption in the event the birth mother changes her mind. These experiences can all feel devastating, but all are outside of your control.

What *is* within your control, however, is how long you're willing to remain on this course to parenthood. At any time and for any reason, if you decide to discontinue your efforts, take an active stance. Avoid using such language as *"I'm giving up,"* which implies a weak position. Instead, focus on making a decisive move to be done. The difference in the message you send yourself is subtle but significant. You should feel no sense of pressure, failure, or loss of womanhood if you decide to cease efforts toward conception altogether. Your reasons are personal and legitimate, and you need to take care of yourself. In so doing, you can start on a new path toward a different, but fulfilling and happier future.

When You Hear, "Maybe"

A pregnancy test result is binary—either you're pregnant, or you're not. However, some women will be counseled that while their HCG (human chorionic gonadotropin) level confirms pregnancy, it is lower than hoped. Expectant management will continue, but there is already reason for concern. In this case, a wait-and-see approach is adopted and a repeat blood draw (usually within a few days) will be needed to confirm whether the level is appropriately rising (indicating a continuing pregnancy), or not. This unexpected extra wait and uncertainty can feel especially cruel after experiencing a prior loss.

Even when HCG levels are within ideal range, some women cannot accept this message of *"You're pregnant."* As one of my patients so succinctly stated after being advised that her first blood test confirmed pregnancy, *"I hear, 'Maybe.'"* Another patient echoed that sentiment—*"Okay, I'm pregnant...for now. But that doesn't mean I'm still going to be pregnant in an hour, or tomorrow, or next week. That's not how my story goes. After recurrent pregnancy loss, I've become conditioned to feel like I'm always circling the drain."*

For this group of women, a positive pregnancy test provides little to no reassurance, no hope, and can thus feel somewhat meaningless. The reality is beta levels don't always rise as desired and these women are absolutely correct—pregnancies do not always continue. There's inevitably significant caution and guard that is up.

The most helpful perspective in both situations is to go back to those binary results. In this individual moment in time, *you are pregnant.* That was the single most important task you were focused on achieving. Hold on to this one moment, as it's a prerequisite for the work ahead. If for any reason this pregnancy does not continue, *also* hold on to this moment. Even a very brief confirmation of pregnancy is a relevant reminder that you *can* get to this point and will continue work to do so again.

Positive News

The reactions to a positive test result can be complicated and unexpected. Although a confirmation of pregnancy is the desired and intended goal, you—and others around you, including your partner—may be surprised to find your immediate reactions are not exclusively positive. It seems counterintuitive that you would put all your time, energy, and effort toward the single most important thing you desire and achieve it, but then not be filled with complete and unbridled joy. The reason behind this is that you know exactly where you're headed.

Imagine you had been involved in a major car accident in which there was a fatality, and you walked away physically unharmed. It would be understandable to feel nervous and scared when getting behind the wheel again. The difference here is that you're not able to take side streets or back roads to avoid the memories and dread of the horrific intersection where the accident occurred. Instead, you're forced to follow the exact same road as you head back into that same intersection and continue the journey over the next nine months. While you may experience some joy from the forward movement of the positive pregnancy test alone, it's more realistic that your emotions will run the gamut and include some of the following.

Relief

If your pregnancy test is positive, your initial reaction will undoubtedly be tremendous relief: "*IT WORKED!*" This sense of relief is fleeting—especially if you've experienced recurrent pregnancy loss—and only briefly affirms that your body or the fertility treatment worked. (The real relief would be confirmation that this pregnancy and your body are going to keep working through the next nine months and delivery and beyond.) The rest of your world will soon come back into focus, and you will quickly remember that there are going to be many challenges ahead, starting *now*. There is little to no lasting relief when you feel the weight of the world on your shoulders, and without an emotional plan to get yourself beyond this moment.

Ambivalence and Fear

After achieving something you desire, mixed feelings and conflicting emotions may now collide and leave you feeling confused and scared.

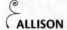
ALLISON

When my period was two days late, six months (or was it six hundred?) after our loss, I told my husband. I took a pregnancy test but left it in the bathroom. I told him I could not look at it. I stood in the kitchen looking out the window. I was suddenly very ambivalent because it dawned on me—knowing I was pregnant—that I had no idea if I could make it through pregnancy again. I was terrified—of recurrent loss, of my own mental health, of losing control again.

Disbelief and Doubt

You may remain in complete disbelief for some time, testing and retesting obsessively, convinced it was a false positive, or a pregnancy that will only result in another type of loss—and soon.

MARNEY

We transferred two frozen embryos, and even though I saw the transfer of them on the [ultrasound] screen, it never registered how real it was again. I left the transfer appointment after giving my doctor a hug and holding my husband's hand tightly. I followed the precautions given to me for the first couple of days, but I remember feeling far removed from the situation: I was just doing what I was told. When the time came for us to have a blood test, the levels came back really high. I told my friend who immediately said, "Oh my gosh, that is high enough for twins!" I didn't believe her, and with each test, I waited to hear that my numbers were dropping. When it came time for the ultrasound, it was on Christmas Eve. My husband had to work that morning and I told him

not to come. I just wanted to get it over with and didn't want to see the disap-
pointment in his eyes. I thought if it is just me going, then it will just be me who
hears the heartbreaking news. Somehow, I thought that would be easier. Unbe-
knownst to me, the doctor came in to check the ultrasound, and immediately
she said, "Oh my God, it's twins!" At that point, the shock hit. It was great that I
was pregnant, but I was just waiting to hear that one or both had passed away.
There was no point—especially in the beginning—that I believed that we were
actually going to have two living babies.

Guilt

All bereaved women feel *cheated by* their previous experience—robbed of a
happy and healthy pregnancy, and a joyful delivery and postpartum period.
Now, through the act of trying again, you may find yourself saddled with intense feelings of guilt, as though you are somehow *cheating on* your deceased
baby: "*I really don't want another baby. I just want the one I lost back.*"

The guilt can also extend to the new pregnancy and baby: "*How could I
have even thought about bringing another baby into this world when I can't even
take care of myself [or my other child at home] right now? What was I thinking?
Why didn't I think through this more carefully?*" Or you may be convinced that
you have already doomed this early pregnancy because of your poor self-care
habits since your loss. You may berate yourself over lack of diligence in the
areas of diet, nutrition, hydration, exercise, or sleep practices—unfortunately,
a reality with grief—even though this pregnancy's needs are very modest at
this point.

ERIN

*We still wanted two living children, but part of me also thought the news of
being pregnant again would instill a hope that would alleviate some of the
pain that followed our daughter's death. When I found out I was pregnant
again four months after she died, I expected some sort of relief and that is not*

what I experienced. The news of another potential baby only made me miss my daughter more, and I felt an immediate and intense amount of guilt. How could I even be thinking about another pregnancy—let alone be pregnant—when my daughter just died? I've had a tough time separating the potential of another child with the loss of my daughter. I know that these are two separate people with two separate stories, but they continue to feel much intertwined, which makes everything about this pregnancy more complicated. Every emotion has a flipside. What joy and hope I have experienced so far throughout this pregnancy is countered with grief and fear, but I have to keep trying to move forward—there is no alternative but to keep going and continue to learn how to manage the conflicting emotions.

Anxiety, Panic, and Even Regret

Some women have a powerful, adverse reaction to a positive pregnancy test, questioning why they were trying so hard to conceive when this good news doesn't necessarily feel any better. Sometimes it can cause women to temporarily feel worse due to the onset of sadness, missing their deceased baby, or guilt over creating another life.

Early thoughts about initial attachment and bonding—or lack thereof—can also surface and create pressure: *"I know I will never love another baby as much as the one I lost. Why am I even trying? Will I now have one dead baby . . . and one messed-up one?"* These statements can sound harsh but are honest reactions from some women.

LIA

Positive pregnancy test. Oh, fuck. Fuck! FUCK! What was I thinking?! I am so not ready for this. I feel like I'm going to vomit. I feel like a ticking time bomb, waiting for the next bad thing to happen, to go horribly wrong. The sensation is feeling like I'm in real and serious danger. How am I going to live like this for months? I never thought that I would be in the position to consider termination [of pregnancy], but I have to admit it's already crossed my mind. I know

*that's crazy, but I honestly don't know if I can live like this. I AM ABSOLUTELY
TERRIFIED.*

Emptiness

Some women find themselves disappointed and confused when feelings of
hope don't automatically follow a positive pregnancy test. Women have de-
scribed feeling *"still dead inside," "hollow," "aching,"* and *"raw."* These emotions
are more reflective of continuing grief than about an early pregnancy. Having
any of these reactions may leave you feeling confused and unsettled when you
realize how hard you've been working for something that isn't generating the
positive feeling you anticipated. Although this reaction is generally temporary, it can feel overwhelming.

Cautious Optimism

Although still sad and grieving, some women immediately feel hopeful about
the future. The term that most accurately and honestly describes this reaction
is "cautious optimism." You know the road ahead is a long one, and the trauma
of the past has made you aware that a negative event/outcome could be lurk-
ing just around the corner. Yet, you are still allowing yourself to feel good or
optimistic.

TABITHA

*We got pregnant again the first month we tried! It was exciting and terrifying
all in one. We were glad that we didn't have to experience the feelings of failure and more loss, and were relieved to know that my body worked, and that
maybe things would go the way we had planned this time. But we were terrified
because we didn't want anything to go wrong during this pregnancy—we could
not handle that. I often had mixed emotions of sadness and guilt because I
felt bad being excited for another baby and felt even worse knowing that the
new baby would never get to meet his/her big sister. But we make a very conscious effort to include our [deceased] daughter in everything we do (birthdays,*

holidays, anniversaries, etc.). It helps us because, from the moment we got preg-

nant again, we knew that the new baby would know about and come to love

his big sister.

Excitement

Some women experience true excitement, even though there will be linger-ing sadness from the past. This emotion may be difficult to access, but it's not impossible. If you feel it, embrace it fully. Your excitement does not suggest that you're somehow in denial about all the challenges that lie ahead. It sim-ply means that, in this one moment, you found some happiness. Hold onto that dearly. It's been a long time and you deserve to feel as much joy as you can find.

LIV

The absolute worst has already happened. So today, while I have this moment, I'm going to live it. I'm going to celebrate it! Then, whatever happens, happens. I know better than anyone tomorrow isn't guaranteed. The sadness I feel will last forever, but I need to honor my [deceased] daughter by living the best and fullest life I can for both of us now. I have worked SO hard to get to this point, and I am going to embrace it with everything I have and am. I am going to celebrate this moment and share it. Life is too short to miss this just because I'm sad. This pregnancy is here today and I'm not going to let anything take a single second away from that. I'm happy and excited . . . and more hopeful than you can believe. You see, if this baby lives, I want to be able to tell her or him about the pregnancy. It's a pretty shitty story to say, "There was no joy. There was no excitement. There was no celebration." Because there should be. This is a big deal.

As with a negative pregnancy test, many women can also benefit from counseling when the result is positive. Counseling can help you process your reactions, regulate your emotions, and improve your ability to tolerate stress and uncertainty.

Whether the result is negative or positive, you are apt to feel turmoil, the Sturm und Drang. And either way, you're going keep moving toward your goal of having a baby. If your test was negative, you're soon going to figure out a way to try again during an upcoming window of opportunity. And, if your test was positive, regardless of your emotional reactions, you've just completed a significant first step toward your ultimate desired outcome.

Mount Kilimanjaro is Africa's highest mountain, located in northern Tanzania. For an amateur mountain climber standing at the base of this mountain, looking up and preparing to climb can feel daunting. This vertical view doesn't motivate all climbers; instead, it can overwhelm them, especially when the destination lies 19,341 feet above. Most trekkers do well to focus on what is directly in front of them, identifying a single handhold and foothold, over and over again. There can be dangerous conditions affecting the climb, including inclement weather and the risk of altitude sickness. Pacing oneself becomes critical. Taking the time to adjust and acclimate increases the chance of success in reaching the summit peak. When trekkers avoid looking too far above or below and focus on what's straight ahead, each step, each move becomes safer, and more realistic.

Receiving confirmation of early pregnancy is that first handhold in your personal climb. ALL bereaved women approach a subsequent pregnancy feeling uncertain and afraid. But that doesn't mean they can't climb. It means they do well to pause here, take a deep breath, and then focus on the next step, the next handhold, and then foothold. That approach will better serve you than focusing on a destination that is not yet visible to you. Naturally, you're going to have difficulty seeing, and believing. Now isn't the time for either, as our minds often give up before our bodies do. Now is the time to hang on, and prepare to take the next steps of your climb.

ৡ 6 ৡ

The First Trimester (Weeks 1–12)

ONCE PREGNANCY IS CONFIRMED, THE focus shifts from getting pregnant to staying pregnant. Anxiety symptoms dominate early pregnancy in the form of fear and worry. No matter when your previous pregnancy and loss occurred, that experience will be your frame of reference for the current pregnancy and place you on high alert. And your baseline worry about the health and viability of this pregnancy is further heightened by something that also affects every pregnant woman—the increased risk of miscarriage during the first trimester.

While trying to become pregnant, you were distracted by the pursuit of conception, which presented something actionable for you *to do*. Now that you've achieved that goal, there's little else you can do to further support this early pregnancy physically, other than take your daily prenatal vitamin and follow your physician's recommendations as advised at prenatal appointments. The attention turns now from your physical health to your mental and emotional health as you contemplate, *"How am I going to manage the ever-present threat of loss during this trimester?"*

To cope with this concern and tackle the other challenges of your first trimester and beyond, you need to gain some perspective on the possibility of reactivated trauma from your loss, and also anxiety. The more you understand your strong reactions to this pregnancy, the better you will be able to manage them and avoid getting stuck during this time of new and ever-changing stress.

A NEW PREGNANCY CAN REACTIVATE PRIOR TRAUMA

It is both normal and natural for people to feel distressed and afraid after experiencing, witnessing, or even being indirectly exposed to some type of terrifying trauma or extreme event that threatened or involved serious injury or death. Fear triggers the body into a "fight, flight, or freeze" response that can protect us from danger or harm during the event. Over time, and with growing distance from that acute incident, fear begins to diminish, and most people return to a normal state of mind that includes a sense of safety and security.

> ### THE TRAUMA OF RECURRENT PREGNANCY LOSS
>
> If you've experienced recurrent pregnancy loss, there can be even more triggers, as you've had more disappointments and setbacks. And, because of your circumstances, you've had little to no time for that activated startle response to calm and settle. When you find yourself triggered, try to use that as an alert, and remind yourself of all you've traversed to get to this point. Yes, you're scared. But your history and experience provide valuable evidence that you possess the resilience and determination needed to continue forging ahead.

In your case, however, intense feelings of fear and helplessness can reactivate as you approach with caution the same places and time frames in which your previous tragedy occurred. The mere fact that you are pregnant again opens old wounds and can make it very difficult to keep in balance with the positive parts of being pregnant again.

ALLISON

My fear was not reduced by my first prenatal visit, where an ultrasound was done even before meeting the doctor. With no comforting words or even a history taken, I was thrust into an ultrasound room. Though it was a different

ultrasound room than with my loss, it felt just like the one where my life had
forever changed, where my heart had forever broken.
And there, on the ultrasound, were TWO.
My subsequent pregnancy included the adventure of spontaneous twins.
Ultrasounds every 4 weeks, then recommended for every two weeks in the third
trimester. Extra scans. Scan, scan, scan . . . more follow up and more follow up.
I went into absolute and utter hiding and told no one of my pregnancy.

Being pregnant again is wonderful, and this pregnancy confirms you were
not paralyzed by your past loss and trauma as you have taken steps beyond
both. However, during this first trimester, you may be challenged to keep your
reactivated trauma reactions from paralyzing you now, even though you remain scared.

Think about a turtle with its retractable neck. When there is a threat of
danger, the turtle can pull its head under its protective shell in an adaptive
and potent defense move. However, maintaining that position indefinitely,
besides protecting itself from the outside environment, would also prevent
the turtle from meeting its own basic needs. It would be cut off from nutrition
and hydration and at risk of starvation, dehydration, and ultimately, death.
The key for you here is to not pull yourself into your emotional shell, but to
acknowledge that you are afraid and that you can use your growing awareness
and understanding of your reactions to move through and then beyond them.

ACUTE STRESS DISORDER (ASD) AND POST-TRAUMATIC STRESS DISORDER (PTSD)

As I mentioned in Chapter 1, sometimes people have trouble returning to
their baseline state of functioning after experiencing or witnessing a traumatic
event, and are diagnosed with acute stress disorder (ASD) or post-traumatic

(continues)

(continued)

stress disorder (PTSD). Both of these diagnoses are increasingly being considered following perinatal loss.

Acute stress disorder is a short-term psychological condition characterized by the development of anxiety and dissociative symptoms in response to a traumatic event that lasts at least two days but no longer than four weeks (after that duration, PTSD is considered).

Post-traumatic stress disorder can develop in any person of any age following a traumatic event. It is twice more likely to occur in women than in men. The onset of symptoms generally occurs within three months, but sometimes can begin years afterward. Persons with PTSD experience strong anxiety and intense recurring emotional and physical reactions when memories of the event are triggered and reexperienced, and even after the initial event has long passed.

Both conditions present additional challenges during a subsequent pregnancy and should be taken seriously. The strategies suggested here can help manage reactivated trauma and anxiety symptoms, but do not take the place of professional treatment, something I highly recommend in both cases.

LEARNING TO DIFFERENTIATE BETWEEN
HEALTHY FEAR AND UNHEALTHY WORRY

Although your history has taught you there is a real reason to be afraid, *fear* is altogether different from *worry*, and many people confuse these two types of anxieties. You'll need to differentiate between them in order to relieve yourself of anxiety or at least lessen it, as each of these two requires different tactics to calm and quiet them.

Fear is the healthy and adaptive response to an actual threat or danger and is something that prompts action. While highly uncomfortable, fear can spur you in *actionable* and important directions. Fear can motivate you to become more informed, cautious, assertive, diligent, and vigilant, even when you're still afraid and uncertain. For example, if you are concerned about the health and well-being of this pregnancy, your fear can motivate you to do something actionable, for example, take your prenatal vitamin daily so you can best support this baby's healthy development.

Worry, on the other hand, creates similar discomfort and stress, but not in any way positive. Worry is a maladaptive attempt to resolve anxiety, but ends up maintaining—or even worsening—anxiety when there is no immediate danger or identifiable problem that you can act upon. Your concern about miscarriage, for example, is something that may, or may not, happen. Although there is an increased risk for loss during the first trimester, there is nothing concrete or *actionable* you can do right now to guard against that. Worry has an insatiable hunger and will look for something to feed on, but there is nothing that can satisfy it.

Consider this example: If you're sitting on a beach and dark storm clouds begin to approach, along with a clap of thunder and raindrops, *fear* can spur you into action to gather your blanket and belongings and head for shelter. However, if you're sitting on a beach and the sky is blue and filled with sunshine, you may *worry* about the threat of a possible thunderstorm, but in the moment, there is not a single actionable thing for you to do to ward that off. Sure, you can leave the beach, but by doing so, you're feeding the worry (which doesn't have *any* impact on a thunderstorm), and you'll miss out on a potentially fun afternoon in the sun and sand.

So, when inevitable anxieties surface, acknowledge them, and then ask yourself, *"Is there an immediate threat or identifiable problem in front of me RIGHT NOW?"* And, if yes, ask yourself, *"Is there anything concrete or actionable that I can do to enhance my sense of safety and well-being?"* If yes, that's fear and you can act on it. If no, that's worry, and you can't do anything to change the felt threat. Instead, recognize there is nothing you can do with that worry, so instead of trying to satiate it, starve it. One way to accomplish this is by visualizing a small backpack you're planning to carry on a day-long hike. You only want to include necessities, such as water and food, not those that just add weight. Continue to assess what you allow in. Focus on things that have the power to aid you in some way and that you can impact or influence. Practice focusing on the backpack image whenever these emotions arise, and keep these differences and perspectives in mind as you encounter the specific challenges of this trimester.

IF UNCHECKED OR UNTREATED, WORRIES CAN BLEED OVER INTO ANY AREA

Your history may have created a heightened state of vulnerability that may also extend beyond fertility and reproductive health where a headache may be believed to be an undiagnosed brain tumor, and a partner's return home from work fifteen minutes later than expected due to heavy traffic may cause you panic, envisioning a major motor vehicle accident. These terrible and catastrophic thoughts can lessen with time and certainly with treatment, but serve to underscore the intense and pervasive nature of trauma surrounding perinatal loss. Cognitive behavioral therapy (CBT) can help identify these irrational thoughts or cognitive distortions and can be very effective in arming you with concrete strategies to change this inner narrative. (For more on CBT, see page 111.)

NAVIGATING THE THREE FIRST TRIMESTER CHALLENGES— CHALLENGE ONE: HANDLING FLASHBACKS, NIGHTMARES, AND DISSOCIATIONS

Like grief, reactivated trauma responses are highly individual and will occur with varying frequency and intensity. Remembering and reliving your prior loss is unavoidable, and will likely include some distressing thoughts and images. You may experience flashbacks, nightmares, and some dissociations; that is, a sense of detachment from yourself, your surroundings, or your reality. Dissociative experiences, just like flashbacks and nightmares, can run the continuum. In its mildest form, dissociation can be a good coping mechanism and help manage stress. Daydreaming, for example, is one way to cope through temporary escape. But, as dissociations increase in intensity and distance from your current reality (for example, loss of memory of specific times or events, a sense of detachment from your emotions, or an out-of-body experience, feeling as if you're watching a movie of yourself), they can also increase in discomfort, and become frightening, even causing panic. These types are more serious situations and require medical and psychiatric attention.

In less severe situations, there are several tactics you can use to better manage and control your experiences and reground yourself.

What You Can Do:
Know (and Accept) Your Triggers

Instead of wasting energy trying to sidestep the inevitable, identify and accept your triggers. For example, if your loss was diagnosed during a routine ultrasound, future ultrasounds are likely to be difficult for you. That association is ingrained and you will be aware of it when being scanned again. Breathe deeply during this emotionally uncomfortable time and try to create new and different associations that will help foster new and different memories. It's like sitting next to someone on public transportation who is offensive and upsetting to you in every possible way. If the seat next to this person is the only available seat and you need to get to your destination, you're going to take that seat while reminding yourself the ride is finite. As you sit there, continue to practice differentiating fear from worry. Over time, and with patience and practice, you will become better able to do this automatically, and more effectively.

Alert Your Physician and Medical Team of Your Triggers and Past Trauma

Every physician's office and setup is different. Some practices are small and you will see the same physician at every appointment and have some contact with an assistant or nurse practitioner. Other offices are large, with five to ten main physicians, and patients may be rotated among providers from appointment to appointment.

Regardless of the office setup, there is a chance some physicians and staff members will not be aware of your history or lingering sensitivities. As undeniable as your past trauma feels to you, it can be invisible to others at times. Although your primary physician will be aware of your loss history, that may not be the case for the rest of the staff, including front office personnel, nurses, physician assistants, even physician colleagues among whom you may rotate.

Some offices will flag your chart with an alert of your loss, whereas others will strive to protect your privacy and share your history only on a need-to-know basis. Whether or not the staff with whom you interface has access to or is aware of your history, no one will be able to anticipate all your triggers. It is not necessary to share your entire history with every professional with whom you interface, but you can be proactive and alert staff of your increased anxiety in certain situations and ask for their understanding and discretion.

Even if your primary physician is aware of your loss history, it is not realistic to expect him or her to be able to read your mind and know what is most helpful. Don't be afraid to disclose your anxiety and ask for what you need to help alleviate it. You might consider saying, "*I know this is a routine appointment, in which you talk with me, complete my exam, and then listen to Dopplers to hear the baby's heartbeat. Could we please change the order and listen to the heartbeat first? Otherwise, I'll be so worried about whether or not there's a heartbeat, I'll be too distracted to remember anything else we discuss.*"

TABITHA

We were so lucky to have a medical staff that was aware and sensitive to our history. Hence the reason we "interviewed" our doctor before choosing her. The ultrasounds were very scary for us because that's when we found out the news of our [deceased] daughter's condition, but we always had great technicians who were patient and understanding of our past. They took their time answering questions, spent extra time letting us see the baby, or even would go back to something in the sonogram if we needed more reassurance.

HOME DOPPLER MACHINES

Thinking of buying a home fetal Doppler machine? DO NOT DO IT. You are not a trained professional. Even though this equipment is available for purchase, for most bereaved women, it creates additional anxiety and stress, and a false sense of reassurance (if, for example, you're listening to your own heart rate instead of the baby's). Although Dopplers can detect fetal heart rate at around ten to twelve weeks' gestation, they don't always work correctly. You can avoid setting yourself up for additional anxiety by not conducting this surveillance at home. If you want to hear the baby's heartbeat, head to your physician's office. Period.

Learn and Practice Relaxation and Grounding Techniques

There are many types of strategies you can employ to help you remain in, or return to, the present moment. Common and popular relaxation techniques can be incorporated into your routine, such as yoga, acupuncture, deep breathing exercises, and mindfulness/meditation. In addition, grounding techniques can divert unpleasant thoughts or feelings by creating a strong sensation that refocuses your attention on one of the five senses. For example, carry a small bottle of strongly scented essential oil (for example, rosemary, lavender, or peppermint) that you can open and inhale its fragrance deeply. If you are at home or somewhere you can access a piece of ice holding it tightly in your hand will immediately bring your attention to the sensation of touch. Or, you can stimulate your sense of taste by taking a bite of a lemon, an onion, or hot salsa. Grounding techniques can be practiced anywhere and can be very effective in instantly redirecting your attention elsewhere.

Seek Professional Help

With or without a formal diagnosis of ASD or PTSD, individual therapy and/or medication may be of use to you. Cognitive behavioral therapy (CBT) is an effective treatment that can help you learn to better control your thoughts and even change the way you think, which in turn, can help improve the way you feel and behave. CBT targets negative thoughts and patterns, as well as cognitive distortions, which are biased, irrational thoughts that don't have evidence to support them.

There are many different types of clinical approaches for individual therapy that can be quite beneficial in not only providing guidance on ways to better manage anxiety, depression, and trauma reactions, but also in exploring other common challenges encountered during a subsequent pregnancy.

Medication is another viable option, *even during pregnancy*. And yet, many women (especially those bereaved) will not consider this treatment, due to worry about the perceived negative impact on the baby during pregnancy or infancy. If you find yourself struggling to control your thoughts, emotions, and reactions, at least have a conversation with an experienced and board-certified psychiatrist who is well versed in women's mental and reproductive health, to discuss the possible benefits. This will ensure you have current, accurate, and complete information to make the wisest decision for yourself rather than allowing your reactivated trauma responses to make the decision for you.

ERIN

Without a concrete reason for why our daughter was born with a congenital heart defect (CHD), I searched for answers and grasped onto anything I could do differently during this pregnancy to try to influence the outcome. I was on a low dose of an antidepressant throughout my pregnancy with our daughter who died and, against the recommendation of most of my providers, I stopped taking it once she died and continued not to take it once we decided to try again only a few months after her death. I knew that I needed to be on it and that the likelihood that the antidepressant caused her CHD was extremely small, but I had to try to do something different than last time. I committed to staying off the antidepressant throughout the first ten weeks of pregnancy and it was awful. My longing for my daughter mixed with the guilt and hormonal effects of being pregnant again led me to a very dark place. I'm not sure whether I would be here today without the help of therapy and eventually medication. It was that bad.

CHALLENGE TWO: AVOIDANCE VERSUS ATTACHMENT

Following a painful or traumatic event, it is common to instinctively or intentionally avoid places, events, people, thoughts, and feelings that are reminders of past pain or trauma in order to also avoid associated discomfort and anxieties. You may even find that by temporarily ignoring or not acknowledging your current pregnancy, you somehow feel safer or better. This can especially be the case if you've experienced recurrent pregnancy loss. There's really no harm in this so long as you continue to take your daily prenatal vitamin and follow your physician's recommendations.

The challenge is managing your feelings around this tactic. If you avoid the reality of this pregnancy, you risk starting to feel guilty and bad at some point—as if denying your pregnancy could harm your baby, or as if you are distancing yourself from this growing person. But if you don't practice avoidance and allow yourself to attach you may experience the same feelings of guilt! The difference is simply that in the first scenario you may feel guilt toward your new, developing baby; and in the second, you may feel guilt toward your deceased baby. The additional challenge of avoidance is that as the pregnancy continues, at some point soon you will no longer be able to deny its existence.

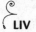

LIV

This was a very confusing time for me. I absolutely celebrated my positive pregnancy test and embraced the experience immediately. But then it started to fade fast, and when I tried to keep that excitement going, I started to feel fake. And terribly anxious. I kept looking at pictures of myself when I last found out I was pregnant. I was smiling, with my hand on my belly, long before anyone else could tell. Long before anything went wrong. I looked at that girl and a part of me didn't want to be that girl again, so happy but so naïve. So, I started to detach. It was upsetting to think that I might go through this pregnancy as somewhat of a bystander, a stranger to this baby and the baby to me, but that actually felt safer than having to have this complicated relationship all figured out today. I also started feeling bad for the baby. Would it think it wasn't wanted, or wasn't loved? Or would it know one day that I was doing everything I could, even though that doesn't feel like enough?

TABITHA

I did not experience many of the typical pregnancy symptoms during my first trimester (nausea and vomiting, only loss of appetite and sleepy) so although I was relieved not to be sick, it made me nervous that something was wrong because I felt like I was "supposed" to feel sick! I don't feel I had an issue with attachment because I knew deep down that even if something went terribly wrong with the pregnancy, it would never take away from my love for this child. I was not willing to waste precious time not bonding with my baby because I know the reality is that it can all be taken away in an instant, and I could never live with that regret. I felt guilty sometimes being so focused on this pregnancy and that it took away from my time to think about our baby who died but I know that she would want us to be happy and to make room in our hearts for her as well as her little sibling.

What You Can Do:
Recognize That Avoidance and Detachment Are Not Inherently Bad
At this point, again, there is nothing you can do to further support this pregnancy physically, other than what you are already doing. Don't be hard on yourself over this fact. You are already doing enough.

Avoid Expectations About What Attachment Should Look Like
Even though it is probable you will make comparisons to your last pregnancy, make the effort to fight this tendency. Every baby and every pregnancy are different. There is no value added by creating more pressure than you're already feeling. If you find yourself quickly attached to this pregnancy, embrace it. And, in the case you're not, remember that you haven't even met this person yet, so it's more than reasonable that your feelings may take time to develop.

CHALLENGE THREE: MANAGING INTENSE
EMOTIONAL REACTIONS

If your prior loss is recent or you still feel wounded or vulnerable, you may continue to have strong psychological and emotional reactions that feel impossible to contain. In the world of psychology, we refer to this as heightened psychological "arousal and reactivity." Symptoms can include difficulty falling asleep or staying asleep, irritability, outbursts of anger, difficulty concentrating, hypervigilance, an increased need for control, and an exaggerated startle response. If so, this is understandable—something unexpected and terrible happened to you that was completely outside of your control. On some level, your reactions are instinctual and some (not all) potentially can help you by keeping you alert and on guard. But they can also hinder you if they're not kept in check.

What You Can Do:

Practice Good Sleep Hygiene

Sleep is a basic need. And, getting enough quality sleep—and rest—is critical to your physical and emotional well-being. Avoid drinks and foods that contain caffeine four to six hours before bed, and ideally stop eating all food, especially items that are spicy or high in fat and protein, two to three hours before bed. Try to eat a lighter dinner and focus on foods that naturally help induce sleep, including those containing tryptophan (poultry, salmon, sardines), magnesium (legumes, nuts, avocados), B$_6$ (tuna, eggs, bananas), calcium (yogurt, almonds, sesame and chia seeds), or melatonin (tart cherries, asparagus, walnuts). Getting regular exercise early in the day can improve sleep quality. If you find you must daytime nap, aim for a duration of less than thirty minutes to avoid going into a deeper stage of sleep where your brain waves slow down and cause you to feel groggy upon reawakening.

Ensure a conducive sleep environment. Cover or remove visible clocks, as they can create anxiety when you don't fall asleep as easily as you desire. Consider using a white noise machine or app. Maintain a cooler room temperature (ideal is 60° to 67°F). Bright lights from TVs, tablets, and cell phones have no place in the bedroom. Establish a prebedtime routine that is relaxing and focuses on winding down rather than rushing to get things done. Try to keep to a regular schedule, going to bed around the same time every day. And, go to sleep when you are tired.

It is important to get yourself up and out of bed if you can't or don't fall asleep easily (within what feels like fifteen to twenty minutes). Otherwise, your body will become accustomed to thinking the bed is not a place for sleep, and that is fertile ground for anxious thoughts. If you can't fall asleep or stay asleep, get out of bed and distract yourself with a mundane task for thirty minutes—such as folding a load of laundry, or something else that doesn't stimulate your mind—and then return to bed and attempt sleep again. Over time and with repetition, you will reinforce to your body that the bedroom is where you sleep. If your sleep difficulties continue, talk with your therapist or physician. Cognitive behavioral therapy and medication (even during pregnancy) remain excellent treatment options.

Avoid Overthinking Early Symptoms of Pregnancy

Every bereaved woman who is subsequently pregnant longs to experience early pregnancy symptoms, such as nausea, vomiting, or breast changes, believing those signs will help reassure her she's truly pregnant. If you experience morning sickness, you will generally notice it begin by week 9, and subside by the second trimester (week 14), although some women experience it for their entire pregnancy. Despite feeling miserable physically, you might also find yourself wanting these symptoms to continue, especially until you begin to feel regular fetal movement. *Just understand that the absence of these symptoms is not a cause for medical concern.* Nausea can correlate with the rising BHCG level. Some women with a healthy pregnancy experience intermittent symptoms, but some never experience nausea or vomiting at all. In truth, the presence or absence of early pregnancy symptoms does not provide any real evidence about the health and well-being of the pregnancy.

Any physical discomfort you experience may further compromise your emotional and mental reserves. It is thus expected that during this first trimester you will have overall higher psychological arousal and reactivity levels, anxiety, and a more difficult time rebounding. So, if you experience early pregnancy symptoms, acknowledge them, but do your best not to fixate on or overthink them. Acknowledge any physical discomfort but don't pressure yourself to remain silent for fear of seeming ungrateful about being pregnant again. That only adds additional weight to your already tired shoulders. Do your best to get rest, ask for help, and talk with your physician if your symptoms continue to worsen, to explore the possibility of a medication to target nausea and/or vomiting that could be safely used during pregnancy. And, if you don't experience symptoms, remember that morning sickness is not a prerequisite for a healthy first trimester.

Be Thoughtful and Realistic About Prenatal Screening and Diagnostic Tests

First-trimester noninvasive prenatal testing (NIPT)—also known as noninvasive prenatal screening (NIPS)—and prenatal diagnostic tests for genetic disorders are routinely offered to all pregnant women, but sometimes create more worry than reassurance.

Screening tests (for example, MaterniT21 and Panorama) only involve drawing blood from the mother and pose no threat to the baby. They differ from diagnostic tests in that they cannot confirm whether a baby has a specific disorder—they simply indicate high or low risk of a baby having certain genetic conditions. They can also be used to determine the sex of the baby as early as nine weeks' gestation. These tests are most often used to look for the presence of an extra or missing copy of a chromosome (including the sex chromosomes). The accuracy of the test varies by the disorder.

Invasive diagnostic tests, on the other hand, can detect certain disorders in utero with greater precision and accuracy, but carry with them the risk of miscarriage. In addition to a level II twenty-week ultrasound, the two most common diagnostic tests used today are chorionic villus sampling (CVS), which is generally performed between ten and thirteen weeks of pregnancy by obtaining a sample from the placenta; and amniocentesis (a.k.a. amnio), which tests the amniotic fluid and is generally performed between weeks fourteen to twenty (although some medical centers will perform them as early as eleven weeks). Whereas many women are desperate for concrete, objective, medical evidence that their baby is healthy and well, others are unwilling to consider an invasive procedure that has any risk of miscarriage, no matter how low the statistical percentage quoted.

Despite all the medical advances that have been made in diagnostic testing for chromosomal disorders, neural tube defects, and other conditions, limitations and unknowns remain. Screening and invasive prenatal diagnostic testing may or may not provide the desired reassurance to you, and may create additional anxiety in the event something is identified and you are then faced with a time-sensitive decision about whether to continue or terminate the pregnancy. Talk with your partner and your physician about what you might do in the event something problematic is identified. If you don't believe you would act if the results revealed any issue, having information about an increased risk and/or an invasive procedure might not be useful for you.

ERIN

The first trimester was terrible. All the excitement that previously came with finding out we were pregnant was clouded by the recent experience of losing our daughter twenty-three days after birth. Pregnancy was no longer associated with the excitement of a future with a healthy child. It could go either way. We have one child who is living and one who is not. For us, the end result is 50/50, so there was no way to feel certain either way about this third pregnancy.

Another factor complicating this pregnancy for us is the increased likelihood of having another child with a congenital heart defect, which is what our daughter died from at three weeks old. Our chances of having another child with a congenital heart defect increased from the normal 1 to 5 percent. This statistic may seem comforting to some, but when you have already been struck by lightning once, you realize that no one is immune. We are at higher risk of this happening again, and no one knows what causes CHDs to occur in the first place, so nothing we can do or avoid is going to influence whether or not this baby has a CHD too. We are going into this pregnancy knowing that terrible things do happen, and that we don't have the control we wish we did to stop them. It's a scary journey to embark on.

Given your history, you're terrified of being in another situation in which you feel utterly helpless. After your being "struck by lightning" once, statistics can become meaningless, and numbers suggest different things to different people. One in a thousand might be reassuring for some, but not if you've already been that 1 in 100,000, or 1 in 1,000,000. Understand your options, manage your expectations, and recognize that even if test results prove normal, you may still continue to experience some anxiety.

Manage Hypervigilance and the Need for Control

Emotions are bound to fluctuate wildly, with varied frequency and intensity throughout this pregnancy. As a result, you may find yourself craving a sense of control. Be cautious of things you think you can control but really cannot, and recognize that total control is not realistic. You may also try to chase control in other areas of your life that have nothing to do with pregnancy, to compensate for the lack of control you feel.

ANDREA

I honestly don't know how I got any work done in the first trimester. All I seemed to do all day, every day, was build spreadsheets to track hormone levels, read blogs, Google symptoms, scour the internet for HCG level anecdotes, worry about imaginary things, and in general, drive myself absolutely crazy. It was excruciating. Each day felt like months. I couldn't wait to go to bed at night so that eight hours would slip by and I could check one more day off the countdown calendar.

LIA

During this time, my house became cleaner and more organized than it has ever been. I alphabetized everything, and there was not one single thing that did not have an exact place or home. I color-coded the clothes in the closets and our towels in the cabinets. I drove my husband out of his mind, chasing him around the house when he'd come home from work, begging him not to undo what I had worked so hard to do. I had to have everything just so. He asked me why this kind of stuff matters, if it matters. Especially the night I lost

my shit when he cooked for me and he put the salt back next to the pepper
instead of the tarragon. That was the moment I realized I was the one out of
my mind. I felt so out of control inside, and I was trying to make up for it by
trying to control everything else, including my husband. Pro tip: That doesn't
work and didn't get me anywhere.

The entire process of pregnancy (and eventually parenthood) is one of letting go of control—over your changing body, when and how you deliver, and the outcome. It continues with letting go of control over your independence, your time, your sleep/wake cycles, and eventually your new baby as he/she grows from needing you to venturing out into the world. Although these can be difficult and emotional milestones, they are all important. The goal of parenthood is to support your child's natural and healthy development—to differentiate and allow your child to become his/her own independent person. That process begins with you, and it begins now.

First, differentiate between what you *can* control and that which you *cannot*. Acknowledge and accept that what you cannot control is of more extensive range and scope. Confronting issues of control is intentional and purposeful work. Ask yourself, *"Is there anything I can actively do or control in this one single moment that will positively impact my pregnancy, myself, or address a specific fear?"* If the answer is yes, then act on it. If not, let it go. The more you chase control, the more elusive it becomes. The more you focus on the things you actually can control (and release yourself from the things you cannot), the more balanced and more grounded you will feel.

Foster Your Entire Identity

You are a whole person who has many interests, talents, and passions, even if they feel dormant or nonexistent right now. Do not ignore other aspects of yourself just because parts of you still feel broken or scattered. Instead, acknowledge and nurture all parts of you, along with this pregnancy. Continue to pursue activities, experiences, and possible distractions (walking/hiking, reading, music, the arts, movies) that previously brought you joy to see if you can reignite a spark. When you feel up to it, you can explore new activities and experiences (take a class or join a book group) that, if nothing else, can help fill your hours and days during this time of wait.

Most important, be as patient as you can be with your currently fragile identity, including the parts of you that are continuing to grieve. You may feel fatigued from the fight to forge ahead through your sadness, fear, and worry. As painful and scary as certain moments are for you now, nothing is worse than your grief. The milestone of your first trimester is a good reminder that you are advancing toward your goal. You found ways to get through each yesterday, and with continued help and awareness, you will find ways to work through the vulnerabilities of today. Instead of having your past fuel your worries, let your past help fuel you. Death did not break the bond between you and your baby; instead, death has proven to you how strong that bond really is and will forever be.

It is this connection and bond that will help you remain focused and encourage you when the path feels hard and uphill. You want to, and will, create that again with this pregnancy and baby—even if it means traversing through flashbacks and nightmares, the challenges involved in avoiding versus attaching at first, and the management of some very intense psychological and emotional reactions. You're back in the game and you're going to give it your all. And, in the moments you feel anything less than that, simply close your eyes, take several deep breaths, and remember that what you once had, you are creating again—a life with possibility. And you, more than anyone, know how precious that is.

I Wanted to Know You

> I wanted to know the scent of your breath,
> on my chest breathing just after your birth.
> I wanted to know what made you giggle,
> when you were sure to get cranky,
> when you would slip into peaceful sleep.
> I wanted to know the mischievous look in your eyes
> that would hint that you were up to something.

I wanted to know what would soothe you,
make you happy,
fulfill you.

I wanted to know your soul.

I wanted to be your mother.
Your mom who would
have embarrassed you in adolescence.
Your mom who would
stand by you in bad times as well as good.
Your mom who would
love you no matter what life brought your way.

I am that Mom
it is just not what I had expected.
The pain coming
all at once.
It is almost unbearable.
I will bear it because
you were worth it.
The small bit that I know of you
I love.

I love knowing that there is possibility.
You were our great hope, our dream child.
I will always treasure the days that I could feel you,
the days that I knew you were alive.
You bring me great hope and joy
still.

—BRITTANY

¿ 7 ¿

The Second Trimester (Weeks 13–27)

REACHING THE SECOND TRIMESTER IS a significant milestone, as it's clear proof your pregnancy is advancing and the increased risk for miscarriage has decreased. Although you may exhale a small sigh of relief, the finish line can still feel impossibly far away. New challenges present themselves during each trimester, so your anxieties don't decrease overall; rather, they simply continue to shift in focus. As with the previous trimester, the more you understand what you'll be facing ahead, the more prepared you will be to tackle the three main challenges of this one.

CHALLENGE ONE: WHEN REASSURING FETAL WELL-BEING ISN'T REASSURING

By this point in your pregnancy, you are accustomed to the routine of your prenatal appointments, but these visits are anything but routine emotionally and psychologically. Many women face increased anxiety as each prenatal appointment nears, fearing on some level that it's only a matter of time until something bad is detected. This anxiety builds before or during each obstetric appointment, subsiding temporarily when the baby's health and well-being are confirmed.

The standard terminology used by most physicians documenting prenatal monitoring is *reassuring FWB,* which stands for "reassuring fetal well-being."

But for you, this "reassuring" may last only a few minutes, a few hours, or perhaps a day, as your anxieties return and continue to mount until the next obstetric appointment, continuing the pattern through delivery. This is especially true if you have experienced recurrent pregnancy loss, as it is likely that at some point, concrete, objective, medical evidence became meaningless to you.

Your anxiety may lessen somewhat once you've passed a previous danger zone, but it's not uncommon to feel vulnerable through the remaining months of pregnancy. Also, the later your loss occurred, the less realistic it seems to derive any reassurance from merely passing a previous gestational marker.

ALLY

I lost my daughter at twenty-eight weeks, so getting through the first trimester is helpful, but it doesn't make me more hopeful. I keep thinking if I'd had an earlier loss this pregnancy would be easier. Like if I'd had a miscarriage at ten weeks, then getting past ten weeks would put me at ease. But then I realized I'd still have lost a baby and either way there are many more steps ahead. I guess there is no such thing as "easier" and I know I'd be scared no matter what. I feel like I'm going out of my mind because the baby can't give me any feedback. I keep wishing I could fast-forward to feel the baby move and kick, or better yet, fast forward to delivery. But then I feel so guilty for wishing this time away after I've worked so hard to be here again. And then not only would I have to be taking care of myself but also a newborn. I really can't imagine that just yet when I can barely take care of me. Yeah, there really is no such thing as easier; this is all hard.

The early to middle second trimester can feel like an odd period of limbo, with you caught between the experience of no symptoms and symptoms. More specifically, you may feel this sense of quiet after early pregnancy nausea and vomiting subside, and before fetal movement is regularly experienced. In the absence of symptoms or daily movement, you may even wonder, with concern, *"Is the baby okay? And, am I even still pregnant?"*

⸙ PARTNER INTIMACY (OR LACK THEREOF) ⸙

Baseline anxieties—fueled by the lack of consistent feedback or reassurance about your current pregnancy—can spill over into your relationship with your partner and negatively affect physical and sexual intimacy. (More on this in Chapter 8.) This can be the case even if sex was historically a source of comfort and stress release. At this point, it's not uncommon to want to retreat into yourself in a desperate effort to protect and insulate this pregnancy from the rest of the world, including your partner. And, it's not uncommon for your partner to begin to express interest in more sexual intimacy, believing this pregnancy to be well on its way.

If you find yourself feeling this way, acknowledge it and let your partner know this is all based in worry and not reflective of your attachment and/or commitment to him or her. Keep working hard to communicate and articulate (to your partner *and* to yourself) that physical and sexual intimacy are important parts of your relationship but that they can ebb and flow during times of greater stress. Avoid overthinking or judgment if you (or your partner) are temporarily closed for business. Be aware of the issue and why it's occurring, but try not to pressure yourselves further by forcing intimacy. Instead, prioritize your emotional connections as you address at a more gradual pace and one you can both agree on. You may be surprised by what feels good in the coming weeks and months ahead, especially if you release yourself from unnecessary stress now.

In addition to feeling nervous, you may also feel helpless. You realize that if there is any complication during the early second trimester, there's nothing that can be done to intervene medically until the point of viability (which, in most states, is currently defined as twenty-four weeks' gestation). This is a lot of emotional weight to carry, on top of needing to finalize your decisions about prenatal diagnostic testing.

JENNY

I had an episode of bleeding at two a.m. I went to the bathroom and was alarmed to find some blood/tissue/something. I freaked out but knew there wasn't anything for us to do. I wasn't cramping or anything and we'd just seen the baby (and had a normal cervical exam) last week. I contacted my doctor and went in the following morning and was checked. All was fine. How is that possible and why do these scares continue to happen to me?

My husband and I had a major heart-to-heart recently about this pregnancy and what we're thinking regarding amnio, etc. Most of the time, I don't think he's thinking about what's going on (because he doesn't talk about it) but he said he'd been up the night before Googling all of these "issues" that they've seen on the ultrasounds and that he wasn't really sure why we needed to do the amnio. I was leaning toward doing the amnio, but I guess I'm not all that sure why, or what I "want"/expect to learn from it. Even with the best result, I feel like there's false hope that everything is fine or that we are somehow in the clear. There are so many "what ifs," and bottom line, what do we gain from doing the amnio? Also, I'm a little concerned about the risk of the procedure (like, how do you forgive yourself if the amnio causes a miscarriage on a healthy baby?). As always, my preemptive anxiety is probably worse than the reality. My mind just keeps going to the worst possible case.

Independent of undergoing a CVS or amnio, the current standard of care for second trimester screening is the level I ultrasound, or "anatomy scan," that is performed at or around twenty weeks' gestation. This ultrasound identifies any anatomical concerns, and assesses the size of the baby, location of the placenta, and amniotic fluid.

A level II (or "targeted") ultrasound is more detailed and only considered for women with a more complicated history, such as those with abnormal genetic testing results or a family history of congenital defects, focusing on specific parts of the baby's body (for example, heart or brain). Both the level I and level II ultrasounds provide your physician with detailed information about the baby's growth and development.

ERIN

It's hard to explain to others how difficult it is to be pregnant again after losing a child. You're terrified, anxious, excited, and hopeful for this baby and at the same time still grieving the child you lost.

Our daughter died from complications from her heart defects, and we were going into week twenty feeling like it was 50/50 as to whether this child would have a healthy heart. The fetal echo revealed a normal heart, which provided us with reassurance, but not relief, as we have learned that nothing is certain until it is. We were incredibly anxious going into the appointment because it decided whether we would continue with the pregnancy. We made the decision ahead of time that we would not put another child through the same suffering that our daughter went through and we went into this [diagnostic test] wondering whether we would be able to keep this baby or have to let this one go, too. The anticipation of another potential loss is terrifying, and there are times I think we are insane for getting pregnant again.

MARNEY

There are so many decisions that must be made related to genetic screenings and testing. Since we did not know at that time what had happened [following the term death of our daughter], I had to rule out that there was any genetic abnormality [with this twin pregnancy]. I felt this lack of attachment to the babies at this time. I remember saying, "If something is wrong and they are not going to make it, I want to know now." I had to prepare myself for the worst again. Unfortunately, that was how I operated: Prepare for the worst and everything else was a pleasant surprise (but nothing I ever felt completely comfortable with).

Genetic testing occurred early. With the level II ultrasound and all ultrasounds that we did have, I had to be very clear with our doctor (or whoever was performing the test) that I couldn't look at the ultrasound until I heard both heartbeats. With our [deceased] daughter, they held the monitor up to my belly and it was silent. The ultrasound of her was still. I had (and continue to have) flashbacks of those moments. I had to hear the two heartbeats in order to move on and only then would I briefly glance at the monitor to see them move and assure me that they were alive. Other than that, I let the doctor or technician tell me what they saw. That was really tough on me.

The end of this trimester and the beginning of the next was when I started freaking out about whatever happened to our daughter happening again. I knew that something had happened toward the end, but didn't know what it was. I felt like I was still very much in the dark.

What You Can Do:

Request More Frequent Medical Appointments or Monitoring

The American College of Obstetricians and Gynecologists (ACOG) recommends obstetric appointments every four weeks, up until week 28. After an encouraging prenatal appointment, you may feel relieved to have a break from returning to your physician's office for several weeks. Or you may find that length of time in between monitoring appointments intolerable. If this is the case, talk with your physician about potentially decreasing the time in between these visits. Your physician may not think to offer something that deviates from the current standard of care. Most insurance carriers, however, will authorize coverage if your physician supports the need for additional office visits based on maternal anxiety alone.

MARY

I told my doctor I wanted to come into his office every day and also wanted as many ultrasounds as I could have. I was serious. Thank God, he understood and didn't act like I was crazy. He just thoughtfully smiled and said, "I get it." Then, he patiently sat and talked with me and we compromised. He reassured me that I could call his office and his nurse anytime I needed with specific questions; that I could come into his office in between the scheduled appointments for Dopplers; and that he could provide me with one additional ultrasound. I knew, at the time, what I was asking for wasn't realistic, but I think his hearing and understanding me gave me exactly what I needed—even more than the daily appointments would have. I needed to know he was there, and that I wasn't alone. I started crying partly because I was so relieved I didn't have to wait another four weeks for an update, and partly because he was being so kind. He did get it. I'll never forget that moment, or him. I think he knew he was saving my life.

SARAH

I think of this pregnancy as one of marking time between milestones. Sights were set on the noninvasive genetic testing, then getting to the end of the first trimester. When we were waiting on the results, it seemed like it took forever for them to call us into the room. Both of us were sure it was bad news without even talking to each other about it. When the genetic counselor came in and said, "Well, your results couldn't be better," we both broke down crying.

Still, there were more challenges ahead as I then started to think about getting to week 16 and then 20. Things that were helpful this time around: more frequent appointments and ultrasounds. A plan. An open and direct conversation about expectations with my doctor.

Solicit Your Physician's Input and Perspective

Actively partner with your physician and continue to communicate openly and honestly. He/she can provide invaluable support, help you explore decision-making, and interpret results, guiding you to focus on what is most medically relevant for this pregnancy. The objective medical information you receive is your best and only real option for some reassurance.

You may also want to talk with your physician about possible travel during this trimester. Generally, this is considered the best and safest time in pregnancy for you to plan any getaways with your partner, with friends, or alone. Travel can serve as a distraction, and in helping you pass the time. You may even steal some moments of rest, relaxation, and enjoyment.

Continue to Practice Differentiating Fear from Worry

As previously suggested, the more practice you have, the better you will become at differentiating your anxieties and focusing on things you actually have the potential to impact. As you edge closer to twenty-four weeks' gestation, the scope of those things widens (at least for your physician). Getting to the point of viability is a significant milestone because in the event something was to go wrong, medical intervention is now an option. This won't entirely quell your anxieties, but it can provide some increasing hope. This is a very big deal—especially if you've experienced recurrent pregnancy loss.

Work to Reduce Overall Stress Levels by Breaking Down Time and Tasks into More Manageable Pieces

Avoid fixating on *everything* (pregnancy-related and otherwise) you must do between now and delivery, or even between now and the end of this trimester. Instead, practice breaking down tasks to avoid feeling more overwhelmed. Steer clear of making long lists on your phone or laptop that can go on forever. Instead, use small sticky notes. This tactic makes your lists shorter, simpler, and more manageable. Identifying your highest priorities, whether over the next two weeks, two days, or two minutes, will help you to focus your attention and energies more efficiently.

QUINN

I am completely overwhelmed, can't breathe, and feel like I'm moving underwater. I'm so nervous, panicked actually, about holding on until I turn twenty-four weeks. Then, my sister is coming into town to stay with us and help keep me company, but even that is stressing me out. And we're also moving in a month. Because I'm not working right now, I'm in charge of everything. The packing, the unpacking, everything. I don't want to complain to my husband because we both wanted to move. We also thought that my having some distractions (and more control) could be helpful. I feel absolutely ridiculous because I'm having such a hard time organizing everything, including myself. It's incredible I used to work full-time and run a company; you'd never be able to tell if you saw me today.

By prioritizing and tending to your responsibilities in manageable segments, you can pay attention to whatever is most important and time-sensitive at any given moment. Think of a traditional Thanksgiving meal. If you load up your plate with piles of turkey and every single side dish, you'll get a bellyache. But if you eat sensibly and pace yourself, you can always go back for seconds and thirds once you've had time to digest what you've eaten.

CHALLENGE TWO: THE COMPLICATED NATURE OF PREGNANCY DISCLOSURES

During the second trimester, your pregnancy is going to become public as your growing belly undermines your privacy. To ensure you have the most control possible, you should be thinking about how and when you're going to share the news with others.

SARAH

I didn't tell anyone at work that I was pregnant; I figured it would become obvious soon enough. I remember being in the elevator, and my bag was across my chest so that my belly was defined. A colleague stepped in and gasped, "You're pregnant." More loss of control. I wasn't ready to share that news yet.

Some women publicly announce their news immediately after confirming pregnancy, unable to contain their tremendous relief or even excitement. Others are more hesitant and keep the news private, especially in the event there is a complication.

Given the increased risk for miscarriage during the first trimester, most women—even those who have not previously lost a baby—usually refrain from sharing any information until the first three months have passed. Many bereaved women feel nervous and wait even longer—until genetic testing results are obtained, until they have completed their twenty-week ultrasound or until they are past the point of viability (twenty-four weeks' gestation).

There are even a few women who don't divulge news of their pregnancy until they are on their way to the hospital, in active labor, or after the actual delivery.

Such delays may seem extreme, but only if you fail to appreciate their emotional and psychological roots. Whatever group you find yourself in, waiting a while before disclosing your pregnancy may afford you a sense of self-protection. By maintaining your privacy, you can:

- Avoid others' reactions, which may include surprise, shock, and often well-intentioned excitement, which may cause you discomfort and conflict with your thoughts and feelings. In some cases, you may feel that the joy expressed by others eclipses your deceased baby.
- Avoid the pain of further disclosure if something goes wrong again and this pregnancy does not continue.
- Avoid reality—something that may temporarily feel adaptive. If you keep this news to yourself, on some level, you can pretend this pregnancy isn't real and you don't have to deal with it . . . yet.

During the early part of the second trimester, your pregnancy may still not be physically apparent, but that won't last long. Whether you or your belly reveal the news, you and your partner will find yourselves again in the position of educating and guiding well-intentioned others.

An announcement of *"I'm pregnant"* is happy news and many people will respond with warm and enthusiastic congratulations. Even if they are aware of your previous loss, the joy of a new pregnancy may be difficult for others to contain, since they want you to feel happy and have something good to experience. Depending on your current state of mind, you may either welcome this enthusiasm, as it may help spark yours, or you may find that reaction off-putting or even offensive. If you veer toward the latter, there is nothing wrong with adjusting others' expectations by saying, *"Thank you for your excitement and enthusiasm, but we're not there yet. We're very cautious given what we've been through, and are taking things one day at a time."*

ASHA

I'm embarrassed and ashamed to admit this, but I'm intentionally withholding news of this pregnancy as long as I can as a kind of punishment to others who were just completely absent and said or did nothing after we had a miscarriage. I know that's mean and awful but I don't want to share this news with people I don't think deserving right now. I feel like a horrible person, but I'm just being honest.

ERIN

We told our family and some close friends about the pregnancy after twenty weeks. This was also when I started to feel physically and emotionally pregnant, so in a way, it felt like we were all learning the news of the baby at the same time. I think this made the excitement and questions from others harder to navigate. I was still trying to wrap my head around being pregnant again . . . it felt like I was playing catch up. Maybe this is one of the reasons I would get upset and uncomfortable when people would touch my belly. I felt like people were touching my belly before I had the chance to connect with this baby, to really feel it move.

It feels like this pregnancy has accelerated some of my fears about keeping my daughter's memory alive. The loss of her and the pregnancy—and this baby—are so intertwined for me, it's difficult to explain to others. It leaves me feeling less understood and more alone than before I was pregnant. Then, I was allowed to talk about my struggles with losing her. Now that people know I'm pregnant again, very few people want to hear about that anymore. I feel like now I'm expected to focus on this baby and only this baby.

While pregnancy is indeed positive, it's naïve to think that makes everything well and whole again. Instead, it makes things complicated. If news of pregnancy comes after the first trimester, or anytime later in pregnancy, many people will think you are home free. And why not? The overwhelming majority of women *do* have healthy, full-term deliveries. However, you know all too well this outcome is not guaranteed.

You may, therefore, struggle not only with your own anxieties but also wrestle with how to absorb the weight of others' immediate investment in this new pregnancy. You may worry about your disappointment if something goes wrong, but also take on the additional worry of potentially disappointing family and friends.

CLARE

My grandmother is eighty-two years old. She was SO excited when she found out I was pregnant the first time, she clapped her hands over and over again and could not stop smiling! She told EVERYONE she was going to be a great-grandmother and was so happy and proud.

It was gut-wrenching when I had to tell her we lost the baby. She couldn't even speak, but just looked at me with such sad eyes, holding my hands, the tears streaming down her cheeks.

Do I dare share this news again now?

It hurt me deeply to see her so heartbroken before. But, I'm also afraid because of her failing health. What if something happens to her and she never knows about this pregnancy? I want to give her that happiness and hope again. I just don't know what to do. I feel trapped.

Disclosures make the pregnancy more real, but can create more pressure through contact and conversations with others. Once others learn of your news, it's common for them to routinely ask about it, unaware how fiercely private this pregnancy may feel to you. You may begin to feel uncomfortable with others' seeming intrusion and growing investment, even when questions or requests for medical updates come from those closest to you.

LIA

We told our parents we're pregnant. They took our lead of cautious optimism at first, but now I'm getting all these texts asking, "When is your next OB appointment?" "Do you have any updates?" "I haven't heard anything but knew you had an appointment this week. Will you just let me know you're okay?" It's so stressful and I want to scream, "STOP ASKING!" I know they're concerned, but the questions don't help.

ERIN

I was in the uncomfortable position of having to tell my dentist I was pregnant because I needed an X-ray. She immediately became excited, said congratulations, and started asking questions. I told her I didn't want to talk about it, and it was awkward. Now that I'm further along, I still don't want to talk about it. I don't want congratulations or gifts or to discuss names. I don't want to buy cute onesies in advance, decorate the nursery or make plans for when the baby is born. Although medically I currently have no reason to think otherwise, I'm not taking for granted that things will work out this time. All I can do is hope that they do.

I have a hard time listening to the well-meaning comments like "just stay positive" or "everything will be fine." It's easy to say that when you've never lost a child. I remained positive when my daughter was sick and she still died. Just because I've had one child die doesn't mean it's guaranteed that the next one will live. No one has that much control. Things happen or they don't.

Regardless of when and how the news of your pregnancy becomes public, you can't predict how others' reactions will make you feel until you are in the moment. If you feel joy or find others' excitement contagious, run with it, and enjoy every single second. However, if you wind up feeling cautious or guarded, be honest. Acknowledge the enthusiasm, but add: *"Even though we have shared news of this pregnancy, privacy continues to be most helpful. I'll let you know when we have another update to share."*

Feelings of guilt may also resurface around the time of disclosures. For example, if you feel happy and excited about this pregnancy, that may trigger feelings of guilt toward your deceased baby. Alternatively, you may have been considerably more excited about your last pregnancy and now feel guilty about not feeling the same way this time around. Understand that guilt can overwhelm your already full head and heart. Do your best to view each pregnancy and baby as wanted and desired, but still different. Recognize the potential for you to hold conflicting thoughts and feelings simultaneously, and that feeling positive toward one baby takes *nothing* away from the other.

A final tip on disclosures: Do not pressure yourself to share the news of your pregnancy in the way you did it previously. And don't feel you must tell both sides of the family and all sets of friends simultaneously. Instead, be selective. Share the news with people you choose and not because you're feeling obligated or you think someone expects to know. If someone in your inner circle becomes upset because they weren't one of the first to know, that's on them. Focus instead on sharing your news with people who will be grateful and respectful of your having confided in them, and those who will provide you with genuine support rather than more stress.

CHALLENGE THREE: THE PROBLEM WITH LEARNING YOUR BABY'S SEX

You and your partner may decide to learn the baby's sex during your pregnancy instead of opting for a later surprise. Given your history, surprises may no longer be fun, and you may wish for more time to adjust to whoever this baby is, versus waiting to learn if you're having a boy or a girl until the moment of delivery. Regardless of when you find out, you're quickly going to learn that this knowledge can become a real problem. After losing a baby, having another one—*whether that child is a girl or a boy*—is difficult.

In general, most pregnant women feel some partiality about sex and might experience disappointment if their preference for a girl or boy is not realized. Pregnant bereaved women are no different. What is different, however, is that there's a greater chance that nonbereaved women will honestly admit these feelings and accept any disappointment long before delivery. Bereaved women, on the other hand, tell themselves the *only* acceptable view is that *"Sex doesn't matter as long as the baby is healthy."*

Every woman wants a healthy baby, but most women—bereaved women included—do have a preference for either a boy or a girl. By disallowing yourself the full range of human emotion (including the acknowledgment of partiality and bias), you unintentionally put even more pressure on yourself to accept and feel good about this baby's sex when, in fact, this is a hugely charged topic. You do yourself no favors by forcing yourself to feel grateful with whichever is revealed. It's healthier and more freeing to allow yourself to be honest about any reactions you do have.

There are two different ways the issue of the baby's sex can play out in a subsequent pregnancy: by chance, or by choice, if given that option. Regardless of how it is determined, there are four possible outcomes, each of which has its own unique set of challenges.

Same Sex (As Deceased Baby) Preferred
Same Sex Realized

If the sex of this baby is the same as your deceased baby and this was what you preferred, you may temporarily feel relieved, happy, and with a slight sense of increased control or traction in your world. Being a mother to another baby of the same sex is consistent and familiar with what you were preparing for previously, with your view of your future life path. But you may soon realize that your satisfaction about this is displaced by anxiety surrounding the health and well-being of the pregnancy and baby. In the event there are any complications during this pregnancy, the familiarity may feel too close for comfort, and you may find yourself believing this sex to be "cursed" or "doomed." In that case, you may also believe you're somehow being punished for being so bold and presumptive to have even had a preference, instead of being grateful for another pregnancy and not tempting fate by asking for anything more.

Questions and challenges may also begin to surface surrounding your deceased baby's personal belongings. Is it okay to consider using the same clothes, blankets, crib, car seat, stroller, and diaper bag that were originally purchased or gifted for someone else? It takes time to explore and process these complicated thoughts and feelings, and even then, such thoughts and feelings can shift and change. The child's sex can also remain complicated into the future, with some women finding comfort or, conversely, feeling haunted by glimpses of what their deceased baby might have looked like as they watch a subsequent child of the same gender grow. Over time, a bereaved mother may also wonder if, on some level, she really was trying to replace or replicate her deceased baby, or perhaps the experience of raising a child of a specific sex. These thoughts may surface and swirl in your head as you realize that while you did get what you wanted, on a deep level, you ultimately didn't.

Opposite Sex Realized

If this baby's sex is different from that of your deceased baby, and this was not what you preferred, you may experience considerable disappointment and feelings of frustration and helplessness. This disappointment only adds more to the growing loss tally. Your desire to repeat your previous experience of carrying or caring for a baby of the same sex may have partly been based on familiarity alone. You may find yourself feeling guilty, embarrassed, and petty for being so focused on your baby's sex. While you know intellectually that sex doesn't matter, that knowledge doesn't make your feelings any easier to reconcile. This news may arouse feelings of insecurity and inadequacy, with you doubting your ability to competently care for someone of a different sex, even though this is not a rational concern. Further, you may feel worried about potentially losing the opportunity to ever parent a baby of the same sex again.

Opposite Sex (Than Deceased Baby) Preferred
Opposite Sex Realized

If this baby's sex is different from that of your deceased baby, and that was what you preferred, you may initially feel relieved, happy, and an increased sense of control. You may also feel comforted that by having a baby of a different sex, your deceased baby's place is more protected and secured with others less inclined to think of this baby as a replacement. However, those initial reactions may soon be overshadowed by feelings of guilt for wanting something (someone) different, and these feelings may retrigger or intensify your grief. You may also develop irrational but growing feelings of insecurity and inadequacy over your ability to competently parent a child of the opposite sex. Further, you may be surprised to realize that a large part of your preference was unconsciously based on wanting an entirely different experience than before. (This is one reason that many bereaved women ultimately change physicians with a subsequent pregnancy.) This subset of women may feel delayed disappointment as they become more aware that they were hopeful for a different sex; not because they truly wanted a boy or a girl, but because they wanted a completely different experience altogether. There is no guarantee, however, that a different sex will guarantee a different outcome, so while you may get the girl or boy you wanted, this may not provide as much comfort or peace as you hoped. Lastly, even with your preference realized, on some level, you may worry you may never parent a baby of the same sex again.

Same Sex Realized

If the sex of this baby is the same as your deceased baby and the opposite sex was what you preferred, you may feel extraordinary disappointment because this is yet another example of you not getting what you wanted. You may have wanted and needed things to be different, but now, many of the same psychological and emotional challenges as previously outlined come into play.

The reality of disappointment surrounding the baby's sex has the potential to be emotionally charged for many bereaved women. Even when preference is realized, reactions can be complex and mount on existing grief, adding more weight to the heavy burden you may already be carrying. Regardless of how the sex card is dealt, at some point, you may feel anger and resentment toward this new baby and a temporary inability to attach, simply because he or she is not your deceased baby.

Learning whether this baby is a girl or a boy can make your pregnancy more real and more personal—neither of which you may want right now. However, it can also afford you more time to explore, process, and adjust to your reactions in advance of delivery.

TABITHA

We had our ultrasound tech write down the baby's sex in a card, and then we took the card to a bakery and had them fill the inside with either blue or pink frosting. We found out later that night that we were having a boy! I had suspected it was a boy and I think I was relieved because I just wanted something completely separate from the things we associated with our [deceased] daughter. I liked the idea of having pink and girly bows be something just for her. I knew it would be a little easier shopping and registering for boy stuff, too. I think I would have cried my eyes out, picking out all the girly things that COULD HAVE been hers.

We chose to tell our family the gender on Thanksgiving by using cake pops that had blue cake inside. It was a tough choice deciding if we should do a big exciting reveal or something low key. We knew something fun like this would inevitably make people over-the-top excited and enthusiastic. But I had been waiting since our first pregnancy to make a big gender reveal . . . and never had the chance to do it, until now. This baby is just as important as our first, and we are just as excited for him, so he deserves it.

MARNEY

When we got the call from the genetic counselors, we wanted to know the sex of our twins. I had to know in advance if we were having another girl or if that was never to happen again. "Two healthy boys" was the news we heard. Of course, I was beyond excited to know they were healthy, but I did have to sit back and reflect on what that meant for our family's future because what we had planned for our daughter's future was never going to happen. We were looking at a new path.

ERIN

Our oldest is a boy, and I got used to the idea of having a boy and girl. For twenty-three days after my last delivery, we had a living boy and girl and that's how I pictured our family. I was really upset when we found out at ten weeks that we were having a boy. I wasn't looking to replace our [deceased] daughter; I was looking forward to the experience of raising a girl. Since this new baby is a boy, raising a girl is something that we will probably never know, and it seemed like another loss.

As the pregnancy has progressed, I'm actually becoming more comfortable with the gender of this baby being the opposite of the baby we lost. I feel very protective of maintaining my daughter's place in our family, and I think having

*another boy will make it easier for me to do that. I worry that others will look
at this new baby as her replacement but the fact that this new baby is a boy
will make it harder for others to do that.* 〜

A new baby is never going to make up for your deceased baby, and independent of the sex, will have an identity of his or her own. Chances are, you are going to ensure that your deceased baby is never forgotten, forever maintaining an integral place in your life and family. You will find ways to adjust to and accept the sex of the new baby and the growing reality of his or her existence, but it takes time and patience to reconcile your feelings—especially if your initial reaction is disappointment. It begins with an honest acknowledgment of what you are feeling and experiencing, and continues with work to avoid self-judgment and projections about what those feelings may or may not mean for your relationship with this growing baby. Individual therapy can also be greatly beneficial in helping you understand, address, and eventually work through your feelings to allow you to fully accept this baby—independent of whether it's a boy or a girl.

THE GOOD NEWS OF THE SECOND TRIMESTER

For the remainder of this pregnancy (and the rest of your life), new challenges will continue to emerge, but you can tackle the ones right in front of you at any given moment, one at a time. From finding ways to hold on to pieces of medical evidence that demonstrate healthy fetal growth and development, to making thoughtful and selective decisions about when and to whom to disclose your pregnancy, to gradually accepting this baby's sex, you will continue to move forward. Although your second trimester holds some challenges, it also has *many* positives that can help counterbalance some of your worries and concerns. These include:

- An increased likelihood you will feel better physically, as morning sickness usually dissipates, and your pregnancy weight gain is not substantial enough to make you feel uncomfortable.

- An emerging ability to experience regular fetal movement, so you no longer need to rely exclusively on your obstetric visits to get feedback about this baby.
- The possibility of feeling more sexual during this trimester and being able to reconnect with your partner in ways you haven't for a very long time.
- Increased freedom to travel (something that may have been unrealistic during fertility treatments or during your early first trimester when you had more frequent visits to your physician's office).
- Decreased anxiety once others learn of your pregnancy and you no longer have to carry the weight of anticipation and angst about disclosures.
- Growing recognition that this pregnancy is not taking anything away from your deceased baby.
- The knowledge that once you reach twenty-four weeks' gestation, you have achieved viability. This is a significant milestone!
- Growing medical confirmation this pregnancy *is* advancing—you have successfully covered more than half the gestational distance to delivery!

You are now proving to yourself you do have it in you to keep working toward what you once believed impossible. Overall, you *are* finding ways to cope through each and every day. Although you may still retain a sense of concern, you are undoubtedly making progress.

One of the incredible aspects of human vision is the range of sight—being able to see in both bright sunlight and in nearly complete darkness. This ability is something most people never consciously think about and take for granted since the adjustment and the acclimation happen automatically. Similarly, in the case of subsequent pregnancy, through natural adjustment and ongoing acclimation, you've found ways to navigate this path forward. Your second trimester confirms that even though you may still feel scared and in the dark, the momentum you have created is indeed carrying you ever closer to the light you so desperately seek.

ξ 8 ξ

The Complicated Nature of Relationships

NAVIGATING YOUR WAY FROM A loss and through another pregnancy is complicated, but you must also find ways and the wherewithal to keep navigating the world at large. This includes your relationship with your partner and any other children, family and friends, and this developing baby. It also includes interactions with work colleagues, neighbors, and even perfect strangers who may have a naïve perspective about pregnancy, or at least yours. Although well intentioned, even many of those closest to you may misunderstand and minimize some of the challenges you face, and overestimate your ability to manage your side of the interactions—especially as you get closer to your due date. Their joy, increasing hope, and pure excitement about this new pregnancy may begin to replace the sympathy they've shown in the past. Your limited emotional reserves, continuing anxiety, and the residual effects of grief and trauma can compromise you and affect all these relationships. This emotional gap between you and others in your world can result in recurrent collisions, making interactions stressful and difficult at times—for everyone.

As you continue through this pregnancy, there's great benefit in further exploring and addressing the inevitable differences, discomforts, and distances that can be felt on both sides of your interactions. The more you understand the various dynamics and perspectives, the better positioned you'll be to navigate them all more assertively and effectively, thereby decreasing your stress, increasing your potential to access true support, and more fulfilling relationships overall.

YOUR RELATIONSHIP WITH YOUR PARTNER

Before your loss, you and your partner were connected and, overall, you likely felt and acted as one. Following your loss, your differences may have been highlighted, and reflective of your individualized grief. It took time, effort, and considerable patience to find each other again in the aftermath, but you did, evidenced by conception alone. Now that you're pregnant again, you've probably grasped onto a renewed sense of connection and unity. However, pregnancy alone will not ensure you're always on the same page. It is more realistic you will both continue to have different thoughts, feelings, and reactions to this pregnancy (and everything else) until delivery and then beyond, although you may be more sensitive to any contrasts now.

Remember, You're Both Still Grieving . . . But in Different Ways

You and your partner are different people—different from each other, but also different following your loss. You each have distinct wants and needs, individual triggers, and will inevitably have dissimilar reactions to various situations you encounter, especially as that relates to your grief.

ERIN

I know everyone grieves differently and my husband's style is to not talk about anything, but I feel like I am the only one who is going through this grief. Another pregnancy is complicated for my husband only because it's complicated for me. I just do not feel like his life has been affected by our daughter's death to the same depth and extent mine has. I try not to let it bother me but it does. I feel like he's trying to make me better—just like everyone else—instead of going through this with me. I know I have to respect his way of dealing, but it makes me feel even more alone.

My husband is definitely more optimistic about this pregnancy than I am. At least that's what he shows me. Our current differences stem from lingering questions about her death eight months ago. He prefers to let it be and has accepted that there are some questions that remain unanswered, while I need to continue to try to find out more. I wonder, though, if any answer will ever be acceptable.

JENNY

I admit, I've been crazy and insecure and made small things into big things in the past. I feel like I've done that a little bit over the last couple weeks with my husband. I was sad last weekend and my husband said I was dwelling and making a choice to be sad, and I felt like he was disgusted with me for still being sad. I went to crazy places in my head (like, "How can we be together?" "How can we get through this?" "Why do I feel more alone with him sometimes?"). He was just being him. He's definitely NOT a dweller and is very practical about dealing with grief/bad things. The next day, he was really sorry for not being more compassionate. I know we can be together and get through this, but it's just so different for us both.

Keep in mind that the goal is to have a healthy understanding and respect for the continuing and highly individual grief process, *and for your partner.* While another pregnancy can be very helpful and healing on multiple levels, it doesn't accelerate or alleviate grieving. Further, differing reactions of varying intensities and frequencies do not automatically mean that one partner cares more and one cares less. They're simply individual and unique. Period.

You May Relate Differently to This Pregnancy/Baby and That's Okay

At the beginning of a routine pregnancy, a woman's life changes with greater rapidity than her partner's, and as a result, her emotional attachment to the developing baby may occur sooner. However, in the case of pregnancy after a loss, it is common to unconsciously delay attachment if you are still grieving your deceased baby or to protect yourself emotionally. In these circumstances, your partner may attach sooner, leaving you feeling upset, insecure, or resentful. This situation can create additional stress and guilt if your confidence in yourself is still low following your loss. It can also create frustration, confusion, and upset for your partner. Each of you may look to the other person for a shared and validating perspective, but find yourselves out of sync.

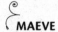

MAEVE

Everything is going extremely well medically. But my husband and I couldn't be further apart. He is ready to talk about names and wants to prepare for the arrival to avoid leaving everything for the third trimester. He told me I can't live in denial forever—do I realize we will likely be bringing a baby home this time around, and don't we want to avoid feeling under- or unprepared? He also said he's tired of being sad all the time and wants to feel happy and hopeful. I do too, but I just can't meet him where he's at right now.

It is also possible that due to an unwillingness or inability to attach, you may opt to lean on your partner and *his or her* connection. This may be grounded in the belief or hope that you will feel less pressure and guilt around *your* lack of attachment. Caution—that's a big assumption about what your partner may or may not be feeling! He or she has their own sensibilities in this area, and it is valid for them to adopt a wait-and-see approach too. It may turn out that they also decide not to get attached too early. If this is the case, you may be disappointed. But recognize that, just like you, your partner may reject the pressure to feel something before he or she is ready.

Focus on the long view, knowing there will be stretches in your relationship where your point of view doesn't mirror your partner's. Do your best to avoid making assumptions, comparisons, or passing judgment when you find you have dissimilar perspectives and reactions. Keep practicing open and honest communication that includes addressing any expectations of each other, instead of carrying a silent standard that your partner is unlikely to meet, especially without any knowledge of it. And remember, independent of what attachment looks like now, you and your partner *both* wanted this pregnancy and baby.

You and Your Partner's Emotional and Social
Needs May Be Polar Opposites

It is not uncommon for one of you to crave more privacy and downtime and the other to be more social and extroverted, not only in times of grief, but also during this pregnancy. This is nothing new as you are both aware of each other's preferences and coping mechanisms—and they may look very different. What you may not be aware of, though, is the increasing potential for you each to pull harder in opposite directions as you edge closer to delivery. This is usually due to a desire to feel more grounded individually and to encourage your partner to move closer to where you are. For example, one of you may try to press for increased closeness and togetherness at home, whereas the other may try to increase joint social activities before the baby arrives. Even with the best of intentions, these differing perspectives may result in misunderstandings, hurt feelings, defensiveness, and anger. Instead of allowing a potential clash to escalate, it's best to proactively communicate your wants, needs, and expectations. You can find middle ground on which you can both stand but it takes conscious effort and regular communication to coordinate. Interactions with family, friends, and colleagues may also cause tension and strain within your relationship due to your sense of responsibility or felt obligation toward them.

LIV

My husband found it helpful sometimes to go out and get together with friends, when all I wanted was to be at home. He always asked if I wanted him to stay home and I said no, but then I'd get mad at him for going because it made me feel more alone. So then, he started staying home more. But that didn't help, either, because I knew it was probably better for him to be out with his friends, and not just sitting on the couch—with me wanting him to want to be with me. His being home only made me feel more self-conscious, and then also guilty because he was mainly staying home because of me. Eventually, we figured out a way to connect by going for a walk together before he went out with friends. This way, we were able to support things that worked for us both.

MARY

I want to skip all the holidays, but my husband thinks we should uphold family tradition and spend them together with his extended family because it's their turn this year. Every single holiday is kid- or family-centric, from Halloween, to Thanksgiving and Christmas . . . and we also have so many nieces and nephews. Even though this pregnancy is going well, I feel like that's a lot to ask of me. We have started talking about how we're going to handle it all, which is good, but even those conversations cause me a lot of anxiety.

QUINN

My husband came home after work today and told me one of the partners at his law firm announced he had become a father again. I choked back tears as his wife and I had both been pregnant at the same time with our firstborns, and again overlapped with our seconds.

I hate that guy. I hate him because he didn't say anything after we lost our baby, which is just crazy to me, when we had been weeks apart in our first pregnancies. How can you not even acknowledge that?! Just because our baby never came home from the hospital doesn't make him less real. My husband says he probably didn't intend to be hurtful—that he just didn't know what to do or say, and that he's actually an okay guy. That's not an excuse in my book.

As before, be mindful about how you initiate communication with your partner and avoid making assumptions about what he or she is thinking or feeling. Be more proactive and direct (for example, with the use of "I" statements), versus being passive-aggressive, which can fuel resentment in both of you. Instead, opt for such language as *"I want to meet some friends this weekend, and you're invited too. If you don't want to join, would you prefer I go out Friday or Saturday?"*

Identify ways you may cooperate so both of your needs can be met. Being strategic about timing can be helpful as well. Advance notice and/or conversation go a long way over a spontaneous surprise: *"I'd like to talk with you about* the upcoming holidays so that we can decide what works for us both before having further conversation with our families. I agree that seeing your parents is important and I can certainly do that, but I don't have it in me to attend multiple parties with extended family. That's not something I'm interested in or feel up for, but I'm okay with you going alone."

Reality check: All relationships hit problematic intersections from time to time, some of which contain highly charged emotions. Sometimes the tension will exist between the two of you, and sometimes it will arise when someone outside your relationship (such as a mother-in-law or an outspoken best friend) says or does something that irritates one of you, sparking an awkward and unexpected confrontation. Pregnancy and hormones do nothing to diffuse these situations. Best advice? *Slow down.* There are various ways through and around such intersections, and occasionally, you both may need to take different routes. When you find your paths diverge, it does not mean your partner is any less committed to you. Each of you is doing the best you can in sometimes complicated and layered situations. Allow yourselves the freedom to make individual choices in real time, but remember to respect your partner's feelings, perspective, and position.

Be selective and creative about who and what you each prioritize, and identify areas of mutual agreement or overlap. If, for example, you are planning a trip to visit family but can't agree on the exact time frame, perhaps one of you travels ahead and spends a few extra days with family and the other flies in for a shorter visit. Don't allow your differences to rob you of things you've historically enjoyed. You may come to find there are potential benefits in some of these differences. If your partner enjoys pursuing outside activities with friends, understand that's not a threat to you or your relationship, but a positive diversion or stress release for him or her.

If necessary, individual and couples therapy can also help you explore some of these emotional divides and identify what you're both willing and able to give at this time. Even if neither of you understand nor agree with your partner, therapy can help both of you find ways to tolerate and accept the inevitable differences that emerge from time to time.

Your Sexual Relationship

After losing your pregnancy or baby, you and your partner may have resumed sexual activity once medically cleared, quickly finding comfort in that closeness and connection. Many, however, have little or no interest in sexual intimacy for a while. If that was the case for you, it may have caused some worry given the deviation from your established norm. Yet on some level, you found ways to tolerate it, justify it, and accept it. Once the decision was made to begin trying for repeat conception, sex might also have been less enjoyable because there was so much pressure and stress surrounding timed intercourse. Or sex was deprioritized and took a backseat with all available energies being used to resume fertility treatments. Either way, there was likely a hyperfocus on the purpose and outcome, not the process, much less the pleasure.

ASHA

We agreed to start trying again for another baby after we lost the pregnancy, but that was tough for us as a couple. My husband felt completely rejected because I would only agree to sex if I knew I was ovulating. I was obsessed with not missing a window and that made him stressed. I had no interest in foreplay or anything besides intercourse, and even then, I wanted to be done as quickly as possible. If he couldn't finish, I'd get upset because I'd feel like we had failed again, placing us even further behind with every passing month. He took it personally and said he felt like he was just the sperm donor. Once we conceived, I was happy, but we're still working—even well into this new pregnancy—to find each other again. Those months really took a toll on us both.

Regardless of what the path to this pregnancy looked like, few couples report high or satisfying intimacy levels after a loss and toward subsequent conception. This is usually the direct result of depression and exhaustion. Once pregnant again, couples often report that continuing depressive symptoms and anxiety, along with worry that sex could or would somehow harm the pregnancy, dampen their interest in or desire for sex. While some couples do resume regular sexual relations quickly, it is not uncommon for activity to remain low or nonexistent. If this continues and you or your partner begin to have growing concern, anxiety, or panic about the impact of this lack of intimacy on your longer-term relationship, professional counseling can help.

LIA

I started freaking out when I added up the numbers. A year and a half of dealing with infertility when we probably had sex four times total. Then, seven months of pregnancy when we were both terrified to do anything for fear of undoing what our doctor had helped us do. Then, we lost the baby. Definitely no sex then. Back to our doctor for more injections, stims, egg retrievals, and transfers. No energy or interest or even time for sex. Then, a repeat conception seven months later. I'm exactly four months pregnant today and there is no way I'm going to have sex anytime soon even though our doctor said it's safe. I don't trust anything after what we've been through. So, that means we have had sex four times in thirty-six months. That makes me so sad for my husband, but for me too. This is so not what we had planned our lives would look like when we got married four years ago. Of course, it's not about the sex, but that is—well it was—a part of our relationship. I'm so exhausted already and, looking ahead, I know I'm going to be even more exhausted after this pregnancy. Will we ever get back to any kind of normal? And will my husband even be interested in me at that point or will he just find other ways to satisfy himself? It's really sad that this is where we're at. And not at all fair.

FERTILITY TREATMENTS AND THE IMPACT ON SEXUALITY
It's challenging to find privacy, closeness, and intimacy when what was once something spontaneously shared between you and your partner grew to include

(continues)

(continued)

a team of providers and was scheduled by appointment, or your partner's participation was not required at all. Confidence and your respective sense of identity may have taken huge hits when you had to rely on reproductive assistance and technology to conceive, even if fertilization and implantation occurred straightforwardly.

Injectable medications can have negative physical and mental side effects, including bloating, tenderness, discomfort, and mood changes, which might not have left you feeling very sexy at all. You may have found yourself withdrawn and silent. You may have reacted with irritability, annoyance, even passive hostility toward your partner over treatments being so unfairly imbalanced, and not in your favor. You may even have been relieved when your partner was less involved, savoring the increased sense of control and autonomy. Although it is not impossible to maintain a healthy and active sex life during fertility treatments and then once pregnant, it is undoubtedly difficult and not at all surprising to see how quickly the flames of desire can be doused. If this occurs, recognize it as a normal response to all of the extra stress and challenge, and also that it's anticipated to be time-limited.

Maintain Your Perspective

Every sexual relationship will ebb and flow over time, especially during times of stress, and independent of loss or fertility challenges. This can be a complicated and delicate subject to discuss, but it's important to communicate with regularity. Remind each other that sexual intimacy was—and is—an integral part of your relationship, and that you will work together to find that connection again in due time. Instead of pressuring or forcing yourselves back into the same sexual patterns you had established previously, explore other connections, including ones that are emotional and physical, and work to strengthen and then build on those. You may find yourselves returning to familiar roles in time, or you may discover something different. Every single relationship is individual, unique, and dynamic. Find what works for you as a couple, and maintain perspective.

MAEVE

Sometimes the biggest turn-ons for a woman have absolutely nothing to do with her body.

I was the woman who said no to sex after we lost our son because I was too tired and depressed. Once we decided to try again, we only had sex if I thought there was a chance I could get pregnant. Then, once pregnant, no sex because I was too anxious and scared.

Then, out of the blue . . . .my husband (FINALLY) fixed the loose faucet on the bathroom sink that had been driving me nuts for weeks, and without prompting, returned his parents' call and said, "No, we're not up for getting together for dinner, I just want to be at home with Maeve this weekend." I'm unsure if I was more surprised by this or my husband, but he just got a blow job.

YOUR RELATIONSHIP WITH YOUR OTHER CHILDREN

As this pregnancy continues to advance, you may find yourself feeling increasingly out of balance with your child(ren) at home. This may be in the form of less energy, interaction, and involvement, partly due to your growing fatigue, or conversely, you may find yourself fiercely protective of your time together before the arrival of this baby. These reactions are common, although either may cause you some concern about the longer-term impact on your child.

Extinguish any negative and judgmental thoughts in your head. You are not doing your child any disservice by being unavailable temporarily and having another adult stand in. Having your partner, or other family member or friend, help with childcare ensures that basic needs are met. It's also fine if you choose to spend every minute with your child, savoring this last stretch of time together, just the two of you. You are not setting your child up for a more difficult adjustment later; you are simply spending quality time together while you can. Children are resilient and your child will be just fine when adjusting to the addition of a new sibling and the inevitable shift in family dynamics. For now, just continue to take one day at a time and focus on what you have to give as you are able, enlisting help from trusted others when you need more rest or a break. This situation is temporary and you will all find a new balance and normal in the months upcoming.

YOUR RELATIONSHIPS WITH OTHERS

As you continue to move through this pregnancy, you're going to confront a wide array of reactions and behaviors from well-intentioned family and friends, work colleagues, neighbors, and even strangers. There's still much going on for you beneath the surface that is invisible to others. While your pregnancy is becoming more visible—and can be others' focal point when interacting with you—many will miss the emotional iceberg underneath. It's not only those outside your closest circle who are unaware of your history and unable to accurately predict your mood or sensitivities. This can even occur with those closest to you who know what transpired before, and may have been supportive during the aftermath. As before, all others around you may continue to surprise you with their lack of predictability, their reactions, or their behaviors in unexpected ways, both bad and good.

Missing the Mark: When Good Intentions Go Bad (for You)

Hopefully, others will provide you with the desired mix of privacy and support through this pregnancy. However, if they don't or are inconsistent, you may find yourself having strong reactions. There are two main ways in which others may get it wrong: when they fall short of providing you the understanding and unconditional support you desire, or conversely, when they overwhelm you by asking for more than you have or want to give, or by giving you more than you want. These innocent miscalculations can occur in relation to the memory of your deceased baby, you, or your complex and emerging relationship with this pregnancy and new baby.

Some people may "undershoot the target." Examples of this include a perceived lack of interest or tolerance for your past experiences and continuing sadness, or an innocent lack of awareness in how you might interpret a well-intended comment of encouragement or support.

ERIN

When I hear comments like "I'm so happy to see you are moving on" in response to finding out I'm pregnant again, it's so upsetting. I become frustrated when I try to explain that grief is still very much present in my life and that this pregnancy is exciting but complicated, only for my explanation to be met with more assurances that everything is going to be better now. I think some people do it more for themselves than for me. I can feel how badly they need there to be a happy ending. But sometimes horrible things happen that we can't fix or make better. Can't we just acknowledge that?

TABITHA

We heard several hurtful and bothersome remarks from well-intended family members that, at times, caused us to withdraw even more than we already had. For example, "I understand. When I lost my mother, it was very hard, but at some point, you just have to move on." All we could think to ourselves was, "You don't understand and never will understand and no, I will not move on. Ever."

We often felt that just avoiding talking to many family or friends would remove the possibility of someone saying something that would upset us or create animosity. That was easier at times . . . but it also meant we were more alone.

It is important to understand that others are not all uncaring or insensitive, but they can have blind spots. Those close to you may sincerely try to appreciate your continuing grief and complex reactions to this pregnancy but may be unable to respond appropriately due to their overwhelming happiness about this pregnancy, or their own residual grief and anxieties about the viability of this current pregnancy. Others may consciously or unconsciously hold themselves back from engaging with you because they don't know what to say or do, and don't want to risk making you feel worse by potentially getting their comments or actions wrong or misinterpreted.

Also, just as your world revolves around you, others' worlds revolve around them. They are going to be focused on their *own* roles and responsibilities at times when you need unwavering solidarity and support. As a result, you may feel unheard, minimized, and dismissed.

CLARE

My mom called me at nine p.m. to tell me that my sister-in-law had gone into labor. What am I supposed to do with that? She knows how hard it's been for me to handle my friends' pregnancies and deliveries, and has repeatedly consoled me on the phone when I've fallen apart. I thought she was one of my safe people, and she keeps telling me she wants to be that person for me, but I don't understand, how could she think that was okay for me?

We ended up talking later and I told her that calling me was just wrong. She told me she thought the heads up and notice before my brother sent out a text announcing a new baby would be helpful. I don't know. I guess I just didn't want them to have another baby before we do. And, I didn't want her involved in that. I wanted her on my side still.

What You Can Do When Others Fall Short:

- **Continue to educate others on your feelings/experience, and articulate your wants and needs.** This is not a guarantee they will all be met, but by speaking up, there's an increased chance that others will be made aware of them and try to act accordingly. At times, you may need to interject or curtail a conversation when someone is expressing advice or an opinion that is difficult or uncomfortable. Be respectful, but be direct: *"Excuse me; I'm sorry to interrupt, but that's just not helpful right now."* You can then indicate what *is* helpful, change the subject, or excuse yourself and leave the conversation.

- **Try to prevent putting yourself in situations where others have more control.** For example, if a friend is pregnant, ask her to be mindful of your sensitivities around announcements and events: *"It's really hard for me to hear about and participate in your pregnancy in ways we once both planned and expected. I love you and want to support you but I'm asking that you please take me off the group text (and/or email/mail list for updates, announcements, and invites). I don't want either of us to be uncomfortable when I'm not feeling a hundred percent. I am okay with text and emails just*

*between us. That feels like less pressure and gives us both a little more privacy
and space."*

- **Practice good self-care.** Do nice things and be good to yourself with
  regularity.
- **Seek others who can provide what you're missing.** You may have
  wanted or expected a family member or best friend to play a certain role,
  but that person may not be able or available to always do so. If this is the
  case, don't try to go it all alone. Avoid shutting down and/or off and instead consider reaching out to other acquaintances, members of a church
  group, support group, and so forth, for their ear. Create a support network, not just a support person.

Conversely, others may increase their presence or participation in your life
beyond your current comfort level. This is "overshooting the target," and may
be due to innocent curiosity, a genuine interest in you, or based on something
they want or need themselves like information or control. In these situations,
you may find that others unintentionally upset and offend you when they
seem either overinvolved or overidentified with you. Examples include asking
too many questions, giving unsolicited advice, or offering comments or comparisons. It can also be demonstrated by others oversharing your personal and
private information with their friends and contacts.

ERIN

*One thing I struggled with starting in the second trimester was how to navigate
the unsolicited questions and/or advice I received from people once it was obvious that I was pregnant. It's as if having a pregnant belly is an open invitation
for questions and advice, and I'm not always up for it. People see my pregnant
belly and my toddler and assume this is my second child. I'm surprised by how
many people immediately start giving me advice on how to handle two kids
and want to go into how much harder it is to have two versus one. I then have
to politely cut them off at some point to clarify that this is my third, not second,*

child, which immediately prompts questions about my second child. Once I
share a bit about my daughter and how she died I watch them exit the conversation without that hopefulness and happy ending that they are looking for me
to provide them. Perhaps it would be easier for me to just say thank you and
walk away, but I can't.

LIA

There is no hiding it anymore. I am clearly pregnant. And, I'm having a really
hard time responding to strangers who approach me and ask, "Is this your
first baby?" Or when I finally had to force myself into the maternity clothes
store and I wanted to punch the bubbly clerk in the face when she said, "Isn't
pregnancy wonderful?! I'd LOVE to help you with your shopping today. Where
should we start?" I froze. A part of me wanted to scream, "No. And no, I do not
want your help!"

I eventually found a way to choke out, "I lost my son." She said, "Oh, don't
worry. My neighbor had a miscarriage, and now she has twins at home! They
are so adorable. You're going to be okay too." Can you believe it? Because those
babies are healthy, that somehow means my baby will be?! I really, truly, sincerely HATE people sometimes.

What You Can Do When Others Overwhelm You:
- **Remind yourself that others are not intentionally trying to be hurtful or malicious.** They are simply trying to find a way to become more
  involved with and supportive of you from their vantage point. Although
  their intentions are good, you may feel they miss the mark.
- **Recognize these are common dynamics in all human relationships
  and not ones you can necessarily change during your pregnancy.** No
  one is going to get it right all the time.
- **Assert yourself and step back from the people and situations you
  identify as most triggering.** Following your loss, you had to be highly
  selective with the people you said yes to and the events you decided to

attend. This time is no different. Continue to prioritize the people and relationships most important to you and with whom you feel you gain some return.

- **Keep in mind that your family may still be grieving the loss of their grandchild, niece, or nephew.** As such, they may feel helpless watching you struggle and suffer at times, not knowing what to do or how to comfort you. But they do understand that this new pregnancy is something you desire, so, they're focusing on that and trying their best to be supportive and positive.

Striking Exactly the Right Balance—or at Least Getting Close

Reality check: No one is going to strike exactly the right note with you every single time during this pregnancy. As confusing and as complicated as this experience feels for you, it can also feel similarly confusing to the people who surround you. The experience for them can be somewhat comparable to encountering a senior citizen who is seen at a doorway, poised for entry. To be courteous, they may ask, *"Do you need help opening the door?"* and then be taken aback by an angry and independent declaration of, *"NO! I can get it myself!"* Or, conversely, they may assume the senior citizen is entirely capable of opening the door, and not offer to open it for risk of offense, but wind up being perceived as or chided for being rude and insensitive for *not* making the gesture. In both cases, while well intentioned, the helpful person still gets it wrong.

Similarly, those around you may act or remain passive, say something or say nothing, and, depending on the day, your reactions may mirror those of the elderly person. You may have suffered in silence up to this time, or else displayed a knee-jerk reaction when someone close to you said one word wrong or made a single statement that was received as offensive or deeply hurtful to you, and consequently has not been forgotten. It is naïve to assume that others can innately understand or appreciate every nuance of your grief and the challenges of this pregnancy. Knowing this will not necessarily help you forget or soften their missteps, but it can help you to forgive them, and possibly cause less stress for you in the long run.

AMY

My best friend was also pregnant at the same time I experienced my most re-cent loss. She went on to have a little girl. Coincidentally, we were also pregnant at the same time when I had my son. Sadly, she lost twin boys at that time. Loss and babies have put our friendship on a bit of a roller coaster. Exchanging ex-cited stories, thoughts, and plans turned into avoidance or forced text messages to check in. It's frustrating when a friendship is so natural and then infertility and loss take that away from you. What was once natural becomes forced, and it makes you wonder who and what is worth fighting for.

People really do say the darndest things when they find out about the loss of a pregnancy or baby. I was surprised at how even the people closest to me said inappropriate things like "It was meant to be" or "Something had to be wrong with the baby." All I really wanted them to do was listen or acknowl-edge that I just lost a son or daughter. And just let me cry. That would be my biggest piece of advice to others who know of someone dealing with a loss or another pregnancy—just listen. Don't try and fix things by giving advice on what you think will help. Quiet hugs go a long way.

In attempting to strike the right balance between greatly desired privacy and much-needed support through this pregnancy, your challenge will be to selectively remove walls you've built to allow others the chance to see and support you in ways they are able. And the challenge for others is to remain respectful and present even when they don't understand all they hear and see from you. Educate and remind those closest to you that active and patient lis-tening (*true listening*, not simply waiting for you to stop talking so they can interject their own perspective) is one of the greatest gifts they can offer. Find-ing ways to walk honestly with someone along the path can be very freeing even if hard. Let them know, "*I hear you even when I can't or don't respond. Please don't stop reaching out.*" In time, they may be comfortable enough to respond, "*Please be patient with me too. I don't know what to say or do, but I am here. And I care very deeply.*"

YOUR EMERGING RELATIONSHIP WITH THIS BABY

Although on some level you may not yet feel attached to this baby, as the pregnancy continues to advance, you will feel increasing societal *and* self-imposed pressure. Whereas some women do feel an immediate attachment upon first confirming they're pregnant, many others do not. Falling in love at any point in life can either happen suddenly or occur gradually over the course of weeks, months, or sometimes even years. It can become uncomfortable and awkward when those around you actively demonstrate increasing investment in and excitement about this pregnancy/baby, if you do not feel the same way.

Many pregnant women—even those without a history of loss—do not feel bonded during their pregnancies, upon seeing their baby at birth, and sometimes for weeks or months into the postpartum period. Pregnancy and parenthood are more consuming and emotional than many imagine, made more intense by societal pressure placed on women today. Although pregnancy and parenthood can be wonderful, there is stress—and even competition—to "measure up," especially when you see other women glowing, or blissfully reveling in their current state of pregnancy and/or as mother to a newborn.

So, how can you weather this pressure? There are two important things you can focus on and remember:

1. Every human relationship is individual and unique. There is no one right way to have the relationship develop or deepen.
2. You will increase stress and the possibility of resentment or anger if you force yourself to bond before you are ready. If unchecked, these negative emotions will catch up to you. You're better off releasing it now rather than allowing it to build and eventually blow.

Ideally, your relationship with your baby will develop organically, in its own time and in its own way. Consider this example: In most Western cultures, intimate relationships generally develop over time with two adults spending time together, dating, and then making a commitment or getting married. When the promise is voiced, both persons are confident in their knowledge of and love for the other person. In some Eastern cultures, however, arranged marriage is practiced and a reverse phenomenon of sorts occurs—a commitment is made by families before the couple meets, and the marriage may occur before they know much, if anything, about the other person. And yet, over time, the two can gradually explore their relationship and come to learn about and care deeply for the other person with the relationship becoming just as strong and as stable as some of those in Western cultures. Both are equally legitimate pathways, even if one feels foreign to the other based on cultural norms and traditions.

LIV

I'm definitely more attached to the baby I lost than to this baby. She was everywhere and everything to me. She had a room, she had a crib, she had a car seat, she had a stroller, she had a smile I'll never forget, and she had a name. I have a history with her which is something I don't have with this baby yet. If I'm completely honest, I think I'm always going to love her more. I'm open to loving this next girl, but I just can't will that to happen. I think I just have to wait.

Instead of forcing attachment and bonding in pregnancy, give yourself time to explore the new relationship with this baby without pressure and the expectation that your love must be immediate and constant. That type of pressure only exacerbates your existing anxieties and maintains you in a culture of expectations. Your efforts should be focused on ensuring that your physical needs are met to support the developing baby well, while exploring your maternal relationship at your own pace. Your promise and commitment were already made to this new baby just by the act of conceiving again.

ERIN

I feel like I'm disappointing people when I answer someone's reoccurring question, such as "Are you feeling better?" with honesty. Am I better? No. I'm still grieving the loss of my daughter. I'm still working through the trauma surrounding her death. I'm still learning how to cope with this life that I never asked for or wanted. I'm still trying to figure out who I am now, because the world looks completely different and her death has forever changed me. I know they want to hear that I'm better and that being pregnant again has made everything okay. But it's not the truth, and when I explain that, I can see that they are disappointed. It makes me feel like there's something wrong with me for not being able to just give a happy and/or hopeful answer. It makes me feel like I'm doing something wrong, like I haven't made enough progress, like I should be more attached to and excited about this baby.

Resist the need to yield to societal pressure. Let your relationship with your baby—both in vitro and after birth—evolve naturally. Remember, you still haven't even met this person yet so it's reasonable your feelings will take time to develop. Meet and spend time with this new little person before making an assessment. It is unrealistic to expect yourself to have an attachment, much less affinity, toward someone who is right now, for all practical purposes, still a stranger.

The path from tragedy through another pregnancy remains complicated for every bereaved woman and those who care about her. The path does not get easier as the pregnancy progresses; it just continues to turn and wind. The same is true with human relationships, which can be complicated and challenging, but also deeply meaningful and fulfilling.

You have already clarified and confirmed the people and relationships that are significant to you, understanding that nothing and no one is perfect. You have and will continue to find balance between the sadness of the past and the hope for the future; between your needs and those of your partner's and your other child(ren); between others' missteps and their comforting words and gestures. You will also find balance between your relationship with your deceased baby and this new one. Most important, you will find balance within yourself. As complicated as all these relationships are, much of the greatest struggle is within yourself—the preloss you versus the postloss you. You can find ways to remain connected to and supported by a community of family and friends—not only for you, but also for the baby to be and for the memory of the baby you lost. Even if those people unintentionally hurt or offend you from time to time, they're still your people and you know they love you.

The real challenge isn't figuring out where everyone else fits. The challenge is working to find *your* place. Your place is that of a mother. Even if you're not quite ready to acknowledge that yet, know that the seat is warm, and it's still waiting for you.

₹ 9 ₹

The Third Trimester (Weeks 28–40)

YOUR THIRD TRIMESTER MARKS THE final stretch of your pregnancy. Overall, you may feel relieved, energized, and even excited that delivery is *finally* within sight! Simultaneously, there may be moments when the remaining distance to delivery seems close, yet still so far. This is the time to recognize the incredible progress you have made to date.

You have not only survived the terrifying freefall and aftermath of grief, but you made the decision to try to conceive again . . . and then DID! You've learned that creating and carrying another baby has taken nothing away from your deceased baby. You've found your love for him or her has not lessened, and it may have grown deeper. And, you have successfully navigated over twenty-eight weeks of serious anxiety to get to your third trimester. These are no small feats to negotiate. Any of those challenges may have seemed incredibly difficult at times, and yet, you did it. Even if you were encouraged and supported along the way, you took the steps, and have continued to move forward. Your balanced determination and mindset will be invaluable in maintaining the energy, encouragement, strength, and focus to successfully navigate the unique challenges of this final trimester of pregnancy.

CHALLENGE ONE: INCREASED PHYSICAL DISCOMFORT

Let's face it. By this point in pregnancy, nothing is comfortable. You've likely "had it" physically and are ready to be done, feeling that in some ways, delivery cannot get here fast enough. Your skin feels stretched tight, dry, and itchy. Your hands and feet, even legs, may be swollen. You're tired because you aren't getting enough sleep. You can't find a way to get comfortable, and the rest you are getting is chronically interrupted by repeated trips to the bathroom. You're irritable, impatient, and sometimes hurting from the baby pressing on you and kicking. You may be struggling with back and joint pain from carrying more weight. You may feel gassy or be experiencing heartburn or acid reflux. The list of physical discomforts can be long and you may find yourself suffering in silence.

Unlike the general pregnant population, you, like most bereaved women, may not feel the freedom to express these frustrations or complain. Instead, you may believe you must only feel gratitude for this pregnancy. If this resonates with you, recognize that *you* are adding an additional and unnecessary burden. You can be grateful for this pregnancy and simultaneously fed up physically and want or need to vent. Third trimester pregnancy is rough. Feel free to express yourself to anyone you trust who will provide validation and sympathy. These physical challenges are real but will soon be behind you.

Physical issues can have an impact on your emotions, too. Low moods can become even lower and result in such outward manifestations as yelling, angry outbursts, or increased tearfulness. You are being pushed to the extremes emotionally and physically right now. Your best course of action is to delegate everything you can to others, ask for help, and focus only on the things most important to you. Do your best to stay the course, knowing you will be soon be relieved of your discomfort.

Most important, be aware that you are not alone in these feelings. Toward the end of the third trimester, nearly *all* women want pregnancy to be over soon. In your case, it's not just the physical discomfort, but also the desire to finally relieve yourself of anxiety, some of which will dissipate when you see this baby alive and healthy. Still, as strong as you may wish for it to be over, you may also find yourself simultaneously *not* wanting this experience of pregnancy to end. This conflict is not at all uncommon given all you have been through and recognize still lies ahead.

CHALLENGE TWO: THE EMOTIONAL CLIMB
TO DELIVERY GETS EVEN STEEPER

Even if you've already passed the gestational marker of your previous loss, the path ahead may feel rough, but *especially* if you experienced a loss late-term, during delivery, or any point after. Although many women find some comfort in meeting these markers successfully, some remain gutted by a loss that occurred so close to reaching or after crossing the finish line.

If this happened to you, there is no amount of concrete, objective, medical evidence that will give you any ounce of comfort or reassurance at this point. You will exclusively be fixated on what happened before, and nothing and no one will convince you that this time will be any different. You'll recall with clarity how despite taking care of yourself, doing everything right, and believing all was fine, suddenly it wasn't. The level of uncertainty and subsequent anxiety over the health and well-being of this pregnancy can feel unbearable. The hours can feel like days and the days like weeks, leaving you wondering whether you can hang on. You may find yourself pleading with your physician to induce or section you as early as possible, like NOW—just to end this cruel torment.

There's nothing wrong with initiating conversation with your physician about the possibility of an earlier-than-term delivery; however, be prepared that while your physician may be sensitive to your experience, there are responsible limits as to what he or she may consider.

Individual therapy and medication remain options, and the third trimester is not too late to consider. Both may help you through this last stretch of pregnancy if you find you need additional support. I once had a patient whose first appointment was five days before her delivery. She was experiencing panic attacks daily, struggling to cope, and had hit a wall. I welcomed her into my office, praised her for acknowledging her symptoms instead of ignoring them until after delivery, and got down to work. While I, ideally, have more than five days to work with a patient before she delivers, we were able to begin to start addressing her issues, which helped her through the birth and eventually through some sharp curves postpartum. Best advice? Don't go it alone. Don't try to see whether you can hold out. Instead, seek help. It's a phone call away at most, and can make a big difference. You have nothing to lose, and everything to gain, including some symptom reduction and the identification of more tools to help you postpartum.

For all bereaved women, the third trimester marks various endings and beginnings. Some may make you feel happy anticipation (such as the end of physical discomfort and some anxiety), and others you may not feel prepared to handle (such as your role as a new mother).

Until now, your grief defined you, and your identity—that of bereaved mother—became familiar over time, even if very painful. As uncomfortable as your anxiety has been for this entire pregnancy, you've proven to yourself that you can tolerate it. You're also aware that following delivery, new fears may emerge, and the unknown of everything may seem overwhelming.

You may also feel as though your grief during this pregnancy kept you connected to your deceased baby. Although the delivery of another child won't dispel that grief or change your sense of connection, it will broaden your ability to include someone new.

Your emerging identity as mother and primary caregiver to this baby can feel daunting at times, especially as you approach delivery. Some bereaved women thus find themselves fantasizing and wishing they could hold onto the uncomfortable-but-familiar physical experience of pregnancy instead of facing the intimidating weight of an unknown future.

CLARE

I keep having these dreams where I'm standing in various long lines of people. Everyone is irritable and impatient, waiting for their turn to go off the high diving board at the pool, or for a ride on the upside-down and vertical-drop roller coaster at the amusement park.

It all looked like great fun from the ground and everyone was pushing to get a place in line. But when it's my turn, I panic and freeze, feeling like I've suddenly forgotten how to swim, or abruptly changed my mind about roller coasters, but there's no exit. I'm trapped and everyone, EVERYONE, is staring at me, and yelling at me to jump, or get on the ride!

I become panicked and embarrassed, start crying, and then apologize to everyone for the upset and inconvenience I caused as I try to climb back down and out of line. Then I wake up, heart still racing, and I immediately begin thinking about my delivery. This baby is coming for real—I can feel her—and whether or not I feel ready, my turn is next.

ERIN

The third trimester was the hardest for me. My [deceased] daughter's first birthday, the first anniversary of her death, Halloween, and Thanksgiving were all emotionally charged and painful firsts to navigate while, at the same time, preparing for the reality that another baby would soon be born. I did not have the emotional space to prepare for this baby while I was also reliving every day of my [deceased] daughter's life, so I felt unprepared when suddenly the due date was only a few weeks away. What if I couldn't handle another child? Was there room in my heart to love this baby too? Would I be able to give this child all the love and attention it deserves?

Increased feelings of sadness and depression are common, and you may find yourself missing your deceased baby more than ever. There may be related pain, grief, and anger over the fact that this is not the baby who was supposed to be delivered and brought home. Feelings of anticipation and excitement can also stir pangs of guilt over a growing attachment to this new baby.

ERIN

There were many times when I felt resentment toward this baby. I felt that he was taking away from her. I KNOW that he is not a replacement for her, but it still just felt awful. Would people still want to talk about her once he was born? Would he unintentionally erase his sister? She was the baby who was supposed to be in the nursery next to our bedroom, not this baby. I now had to make room for another child in what I felt was her space. It was painful to move her clothes out of her drawers to make room for the new baby. I ended up changing very little in the nursery. It was more comforting to keep her visible than to try to remove her.

MAEVE

I purchased a few things for this baby even though I swore up and down I'd never do that until after delivery. I haven't told anyone, including my husband, and hid the items in the back of my closet. The truth is I am attached, and even somewhat excited, but I haven't admitted that to anyone. I need to figure out what that means first for myself, and for the baby boy I lost.

Anxiety and panic may resurface and escalate as you worry about nearing the end of this pregnancy, concerned about something going wrong, the birth itself, and the potential for flashbacks.

JANE

Everyone keeps cheering me on. "You're almost there!" "The end is in sight!" "Just keep holding on, a little longer!" What they can't see is that my palms are sweaty and I feel like I'm losing my grip and that my muscles are cramping and fatiguing out. I honestly don't know how much longer I can hang on. I feel like I have been waiting for the other shoe to drop for months, because that is what I know. I'm still waiting, but the pressure feels even greater because there's a shorter window (between now and delivery) for that to occur.

ERIN

As the pregnancy progressed, I became increasingly worried that this baby would die too. While I should have been excitedly reading about how my baby was the size of a honeydew melon this week, I was focused on mortality and complication rates.

My fear and uncertainty also increased. It was difficult to be around other people, especially because as the due date approached everyone was getting more excited, while I was becoming more terrified. I had no confidence in my

*ability to love and care for this child. I couldn't sleep. I had panic attacks. I
started to cut myself off from everyone, including my husband, who I felt increasingly disconnected from. I felt like I could no longer effectively communicate with anyone. I wanted to escape from it all. I felt trapped.*

Doubts can swirl surrounding your capabilities as a mother. You may find
yourself second-guessing past decisions, questioning how prepared you really
are, especially if you decided against purchasing or placing any baby items at
home before delivery. Time can feel as though it's slipping through your fin-
gers, leaving you with more to do than you have time for, or conversely, concerned that time is moving too slowly, leaving you wondering whether you'll
have enough stamina or momentum to get you through your due date and
beyond.

A practical perspective to adopt is to have faith in the process that has already carried you so far. You have spent weeks and months preparing for this
time. And, you have been successful in scaling every single hurdle that has
been placed in front of you to get here. Stay the course, and keep doing what
you have been doing; it's working.

CHALLENGE THREE: REMAINING DISCUSSIONS AND DECISIONS

Take time with your partner to coordinate any outstanding planning (such as
any special dinners or dates), preparations (for the nursery, help at home, time
off from work), and discuss expectations you have for the remainder of this
trimester. These decisions may require multiple conversations but will help
you get organized and ensure your needs are expressed, thereby increasing
the potential for them to be met.

Here are some ways to make the best use of the time that remains before
the baby arrives.

Planning Your Time and Activities

You and your partner may have different priorities during these remaining
weeks. Keep communicating regularly about what you both want and need
right now. This is a good time to determine whether you will:

- Plan any last special dates (a dinner, a couple's spa day), or even a stay-cation. These type of activities can not only help pass the time, but also give you important alone time as a couple that will be harder to come by once the baby arrives.
- Attend prenatal or birthing classes. If it is helpful, inquire about the option of a private class to avoid being lumped together with first-time expectant parents.
- Consider having a baby shower. Be honest with yourself about this. You were cheated out of the full experience of pregnancy previously and, even if you were triggered by or declined invites to others' showers afterward, you may still find yourself wanting one of your own.
- Think about and start planning for what you need after the baby arrives, such as how much maternity/paternity leave you have, what childcare needs you are anticipating, and other help you may need at home with housecleaning and/or pets. You don't have to have everything finalized before delivery, but it can be helpful to have some ideas and preliminary plans in the works.

Consider a Hospital Orientation Before Delivery

If you're returning to the same hospital as before, this can awaken old memories and past trauma. Many women find it helpful to return to the hospital and the labor and delivery floor in advance of the birth. Requesting an appointment to visit the hospital will give you time to adjust, and your emotions won't be as high as they will be on the date of your delivery. During this visit, you'll have an excellent opportunity to ask questions and obtain clarifications before that first contraction. Create a checklist of questions to ask your physician and/or hospital staff. Suggested items can include:

What is my primary physician's expected availability around the time of delivery?

Will the delivering physician be left up to chance based on which obstetric partner is on call when I go into labor? If so, can I meet him or her prior?

If an induced labor is required and my primary physician will start the
  process, will he or she see me through delivery? Or should I anticipate a
  partner to perform or finish the actual delivery?
What is the process to request or decline the same labor and delivery nurse
  or delivery and postpartum rooms I had previously?

BECKY

As I entered my third trimester, I could feel myself becoming increasingly at-
tached to the baby growing inside of me, and was starting to feel like I might
actually get to bring home a baby this time. However, I could not bring my-
self to look at any baby items, create a registry, or get the room ready for the
baby. My husband and I had created a plan that once the baby came, someone
would go out and purchase the things that we needed. However, I started to
have signs of preterm labor and was sent to the hospital. While we are still
currently pregnant at thirty-six weeks, we took the scare as a chance to get
prepared for the new baby to come home. The bedroom is now painted, but we
are not yet ready to bring anything into the house. All of our items are currently
being held at a relative's house or at the store.

One positive about going into the hospital before the actual birth of our
new baby was that it gave us a trial run of sorts. We learned how to assert our
emotional needs and express our concerns about being back in certain rooms.
We have now dealt with nurses and doctors and have explained what our
needs are. We have experienced the post-traumatic stress of passing the room
where our daughters spent their entire life. All of this has made the thought of
welcoming this baby into the world just a little easier as we continue to wait.

ERIN

My husband and I talked with our counselor about making decisions before
delivery that would set us up to be able to survive and, hopefully, even find joy
in those first few days, weeks, and months after he was born.

Having a child after losing a child is traumatic. The last time I delivered a
baby, it was my daughter. The last time I brought a baby home, it was her. The

last time I breastfed a baby, fed a baby a bottle, swaddled a baby, rocked a
baby, and sang to a baby, it was her. I would be experiencing all these things
again for the first time since she died with a different baby. There is no way that
this wasn't going to be extremely tough emotionally. I don't think I would have
been able to bond with him and navigate those first few days and weeks with-
out having had a well-thought-out plan prior to delivery.

Whether or not you decide to return to the hospital in advance of delivery, be sure to alert your physician of any individual preferences you have so that your requests can be accommodated to the greatest extent possible. In doing so, you will avoid leaving things up to chance that you may have the power to control.

Regarding the Baby

Have you and your partner already begun discussing possible baby names? Or do you find yourself unable or unwilling to go there until after there is a baby you can see and hold? Whatever the case, don't stress over this—you do *not* have to determine the final name for the baby right now. Although many women pressure themselves to choose a name during their third trimester, this is not a time-sensitive issue now. If it's useful to talk about names, talk as much as you wish. However, it's reasonable to wait until after you've had a chance to meet this baby before you start trying out names, much less decide.

It can also be helpful to revisit your thoughts and feelings regarding the baby's room and belongings. You may have some existing items at home from your deceased baby, or saved from a previous child, and it's useful to consider whether or not you will use any of those things for this baby. If not, you can itemize which baby items you will need to purchase and where to keep them before delivery.

If you find yourself unwilling to purchase anything prior to delivery due to worry, superstition, or a lack of attachment, go with your gut. On the other hand, you may suddenly find yourself beginning to bond, and this may en- courage you to focus on some preparations at home. You may even experience your "nesting" instinct kicking in or feel an intense desire to get your home organized and ready for this coming baby. This type of preparation can be satisfying and a productive way to pass the time, but if you begin to feel the rumblings of any stressful or conflicting feelings, take a break. It could be that you're getting caught emotionally between wanting to be prepared and feeling cautious over setting up a nursery for a baby who is not yet here.

Most women find some middle ground by having the bare basics on hand or on order, and dealing with the rest postdelivery. Women who deliver vaginally standardly remain in the hospital for two days; for those who require a cesarean section, three days. You can designate your partner, family, friends, or Amazon to ensure you have a car seat on hand when you leave the hospital. Even if you wait until delivery, you will have two to three days' notice to get everything else organized before bringing the baby home. Babies need very little at first: food, diapers, and a safe place to sleep. That's all. Everything else can be decided on and purchased later, when needed.

Preparing to Announce the News

Do not assume that you and your partner feel the same about how and when to share the news of this baby's birth. Instead, begin to discuss your preferences and expectations with each other now to identify a mutually agreed-upon plan for disclosures.

LIA

After delivery, I remember seeing the baby on the warming table while the nurses were getting her cleaned up. I had a second-degree tear and was in the process of getting stitched back up. Because I could hear the baby crying, I knew she was alive, and decided to close my eyes for a few minutes. I felt like I could finally take a deep breath after months and months of holding it. I started to drift. Maybe fifteen minutes later, my husband came over and told me he had just taken an adorable picture of the baby who was all clean and swaddled, and now sleeping. When he went to show it to me, his phone started blowing up with all of these congratulatory texts. He had apparently also shared this with both of our families. I was not ready for that and I was absolutely furious.

You may need some time after the birth to catch your breath and rest for a few hours before you jump into making announcements. That is more than reasonable. But your partner will also have thoughts and feelings about this, so work to share yours, but also strike a balance to ensure you hear theirs.

Supporting Your Other Children at Home

As delivery nears, you and your partner may wonder how to prepare your other child/children for the arrival of this new baby and its impact. What follows are commonsense ways to acclimate younger children to the pending arrival of a new baby sibling—all with little effort:

- With children of toddler age, reinforce the ideas of patience and delayed gratification. Emphasize the concept of turn-taking and occasional waiting—something you can even demonstrate when alone with your child by asking him or her to briefly wait while you use the bathroom or answer a phone call. By reinforcing these concepts now, your child will become gradually acclimated to the idea of having to share time, space, toys, and parental attention.

- Extend compassion and provide more reassurances. *"I know you're disappointed that I'll be gone for a few hours this afternoon and we won't be able to play like we usually do, but I've asked Grandma to come and stay with you. I'm excited she can—you both had so much fun the last time she was here! I'll be home before dinner, and if you like, we'll have time to read some books together then. Maybe you'd even like to pick them out while Grandma is here."*

- Maintain every child's routine to the greatest extent possible. Consistency is key with little people. If, at times, another adult must babysit, maintaining set bedtimes and mealtimes can help uphold familiar and predictable patterns.

- Do what works for both you and your child right now. Again, there will be an adjustment period for both of you, regardless of how much or how little time is shared now. And, independent of the quantity of time shared, focus on the quality—not only with your child but in all your relationships.

These suggestions work well for young children under the age of approximately six to nine years who will predominantly follow your lead. But older children can benefit from additional sensitivities here too. As children grow beyond the ages of six to nine, they experience their world in increasingly personal ways, focused on how external events affect them individually (for example, having to miss a day of school, or having another child move into their room to make space for the arrival of the baby). Their feelings and experiences are important too, and they can benefit greatly from repeated acknowledgments of this and efforts to uphold their routines and the things most important to them, such as baseball practice, or having some say in the organization and integration of another child into their bedroom. Further, it can be very useful to reinforce you are available and will provide undivided attention to them (even if it's for five minutes at a time). Just because they're developmentally more independent and more mature than younger children, that doesn't mean they need less attention or love. Strive to find balance by practicing turn-taking yourself, working to intermittently prioritize each of your children's needs (along with yours and your partner's), and giving them all extra reassurance that their place is secure.

ON MOVING FURNITURE, BEDS, AND ROOMS

Before you begin moving furniture and rearranging kids' beds and rooms, give yourself a break. There are many schools of thought about what you must do before bringing the baby home or for your other children, suggesting that if you do (or don't do) this or that, you'll create negative associations with the baby. Stop right there. It's obvious, there's going to be some adjustment for you all, no matter when or how these changes occur. For some families it makes sense and works best to make some of these changes now and allow for a more gradual transition (for example, if your toddler is starting to crawl out of his or her crib, it's time for a toddler or twin bed). For others, it's better to keep with what's working as long as possible and have most of the changes occur all at once. Assess where you are as individual members of one family and then make decisions in real time accordingly.

Thoughts of your deceased baby, your child at home, and this new baby may make you feel torn from time to time. Recognize you are not choosing any one of these relationships over the other. These are all important relationships, and you can find ways to prioritize each of them in meaningful ways at different moments and times. Avoid putting unnecessary pressure on yourself, obsessing over how your child at home is going to react to this baby. There are a lot more than just the first impressions—not only for your child or children at home but also for you and this new baby. Remove expectations surrounding those first moments and remind yourself that relationships are built, and strengthened, over time.

The Involvement and Role of Your Family and Friends

Those around you may have moved on from grief and are now excited and focused on your forthcoming birth. You may continue to have complicated feelings around this, as you contend with well-meaning others who may have very different vantage points. Although you can try to encourage others to be supportive and helpful, it's not a guarantee they will be able to rise to the occasion in all the ways you wish.

MARY

I saw my aunt this weekend and she said excitedly, "When are you going to get the nursery ready? This baby is going to come and you have to be ready!" Then, my uncle chimed in, "What do you mean you don't want to make plans for Thanksgiving? As a family we have so much to be thankful for, and your mom just told us both there's nothing wrong with this baby!"

I was at a complete loss for words. They just don't get it.

ASHA

I worked hard to proactively tell others, "Please no gifts until after delivery—I'm feeling too cautious." Well, that hasn't worked so well. The tally is now up to three gifts after my mother-in-law just came over and said, "I know you said you didn't want anything, but I couldn't resist, and this is just something small

*[a onesie]. It was on sale and it was the only one left. I thought you'd love it
and I didn't want to take a chance on it not being there in a month." I feel like
the bad guy for ruining everyone else's fun and excitement. At least I got out of
having a baby shower.* ⌇

Your efforts to exercise more control may cause you stress, discomfort,
and tension, and increase your overall level of anxiety. Dealing with other
people—whether hosting, tolerating, or appeasing them—can be exhausting.
You may prefer to keep your head down until after delivery, only then falling
into the arms of your partner, due to sheer exhaustion alone. You may need
much rest before you even consider greeting family members and friends. Alternatively, you may be very receptive and wanting family and friends present
and involved leading up to and at delivery to keep you company, provide support, and help out around the house.

You and your partner are wise to discuss how you will handle eager visitors during the remainder of this trimester. You'll also need to decide who,
if anyone, will be invited into town or the hospital during delivery and early
postpartum, and what those arrangements will be. These discussions should
clarify both of your preferences. Once some decisions are made, you can
respectfully communicate them to others. However, if you opt for greater
privacy, some people may be surprised or disappointed by their exclusions,
especially if they were included before.

No one should assume that the role they played last time will be the same
this time. It's worthwhile to clarify this upfront to family and/or friends: *"We
are planning to do things differently this time and wanted to communicate our
wishes. Under the circumstances, we'd prefer a private delivery, and to meet this
baby before we introduce him or her to others. You will be one of the first to meet
him/her when we're ready, but we need to get through the delivery first."*

Family dynamics can be tricky for you and your partner to navigate, wanting to avoid hurt feelings, if, for example, your mother's presence is requested
immediately, but your mother-in-law's is not. You may have the ability to exercise more control here and are well advised to focus on your own needs and

wants. This can be a very delicate time for every pregnant woman, but even more so for you, especially if your partner has different feelings and if you're both struggling with what feels fair or right. Any family history of differences between your family and your partner's can quickly resurface and lead to score keeping, which adds more stress to the mix. The pressure can increase further if family members supported you during your grief journey or were present for a prior birth. It is understandable for you to be concerned about wanting to avoid their feeling disappointed or hurt. Don't worry about what may be expected or proper. Focus on what feels least stressful for you and your partner. Having some privacy may be necessary. You owe it to yourselves to express this to others while offering reassurance that they *will* meet this baby in a time and manner that is most comfortable for everyone.

Everyone loves to see and hold a new baby, but it's difficult to anticipate how you will feel until you are in the moment. You might not be ready to share your baby with everyone immediately; or, you might feel the total opposite. Regardless, like most women who have given birth, you will need time for rest, recovery, and acclimation, so try to create the space you need to do just that.

Independent of your decisions, this all remains new territory, and as with grief, your reactions to the remainder of this trimester and your anticipated wants at delivery will be highly individual and not predictable. Do your best to communicate honestly as you wrestle with these decisions and then be specific, clear, and direct with your family about your preferences. Even if you opt for more privacy now through delivery, that won't last indefinitely, so consider when and how you will invite family back in.

TABITHA

We were terrified about delivery but so excited about the possibility of finally bringing home a little bundle after waiting so long. It was not going to be our daughter but we felt grateful and blessed to have the opportunity again. We spent a lot of time discussing what we envisioned the delivery/hospital stay looking like. We knew there was a chance nothing would go according to plan, especially if medical intervention was required for the baby or myself, but we wanted to be as prepared as we could be going into it. And we also wanted to "warn" our family that although they might envision it going one way (being present for labor and immediately after birth) that is not what we wanted. For example, I did not want anyone to know that I was in labor because I knew there would either be endless questions, calls, texts, and a chance someone would show up at the hospital unwelcomed. We really wanted to spend the first half of our hospital stay just the three of us.

Your Partner's Role?

Finally, one of the most important conversations you should have with your partner during this trimester is to discuss and clarify the temporary expectations and decisions that affect *you* during and after delivery. While you are both equal parents to this baby, there is *nothing* equal about your paths over these next weeks, and the weeks and months that follow.

QUINN

I can't even remember how it came up but my husband made some comment about my breastfeeding this baby. I immediately stopped him and told him there is absolutely NO WAY I am taking that on. It was awful before even with great lactation support. I didn't produce enough milk, the baby didn't latch well, and it was all very stressful. I've already decided to use formula this time and I want his support because a part of me feels guilty about that choice. There's only so much I'm willing to take on. Bloody nipples are not one of them.

Physically, there is considerably more on your plate as the pregnant and postpartum mother. Even with a textbook vaginal delivery or C-section, do not underestimate the physical toll of birth and your subsequent recovery. Sure, there will be challenges for you both, but YOU are the one physically giving birth and potentially nursing the baby. And it's impossible to know in advance what support role your partner will play.

Many women idealize having their partner or family with them, but when the time comes, they respond in one of two ways: either they depend totally on their partner's support throughout the process; or the stress, pain, and length of delivery culminates in an outburst of *"Get the f**k away from me!"* You won't know how you will feel until you are in the throes of labor, and the childbirth experience differs significantly from woman to woman. While a conversation about you and your partner is noble here, at the end of the day, YOU get to dictate the terms for your body and can't do that realistically in advance. The best you can do now is consider a range of scenarios that may occur, and discuss how you ideally see your partner's involvement in each situation. Perhaps it's worth apologizing or asking for forgiveness in advance—in case your evil twin emerges during the birth or its aftermath. Most of all, demonstrating your love and appreciation of your partner now can go a long way too.

Your third trimester is another significant milestone, and confirmation that you have already completed the lion's share of work with this pregnancy. That's good news because there is less pregnancy ahead of you than behind you. You don't have to learn new coping strategies at this point—you just have to keep rolling. You may feel nervous, but soon, instead of believing what your feelings (and worries) tell you, your experience will *show* you how capable you are. You may be frustrated by your compromised physical and emotional reserves, but those limitations will also force you to prioritize and see the things that are most important. You won't have the patience to tolerate anything other than that. All this anticipation will soon peak, putting the anxiety of pregnancy well behind you, and freeing you to focus on healing your body and adjusting to this next chapter of your life with this new baby. Use this time wisely to plan and prepare yourself and others for the next stop, which is delivery. In a few weeks, the physical process of birth will confirm that you and your body are not only amazing, but capable of the incredible. In the aftermath of your loss, you never thought you could or would be able to get through another pregnancy, but look at you now.

⟩ 10 ⟨

Delivery and Early Postpartum

YOU HAVE BEEN WAITING AND waiting for this day, a day so long in coming, and one you may have thought never would arrive, but that day is *finally* here! You may feel tremendous relief, happiness, and excitement to have reached your delivery. You may also feel nervous and emotional as you anticipate all the new and different challenges ahead for postpartum adjustment and parenthood, but know those reactions do not in any way suggest you are not ready. Rather, they are expected and normal for anyone facing such a momentous and life-changing event. You have planned and prepared, and your body is ready. You will get through this last day of pregnancy and your delivery, along with the help of your partner and medical team. Focus only on today, on each moment as it comes, and avoid overthinking or projecting yourself into the future.

In many ways, you have been holding your breath for months, so be prepared that any hint of anything going awry—whether a delay or deviation from your plan—can threaten your need for control and trigger an extreme reaction in you.

MARY

We got in the car to head to the hospital on the morning of my scheduled induction. I was uncomfortable and tired because I hadn't slept much at all the night before, and just wanted to close my eyes, so I did. When I opened them, I realized my husband had taken the expressway and not Lake Shore Drive as I had expected! How could we not have talked about this before? I thought we had covered everything. Right now, I really need to have everything go my way. As in EVERYTHING. As I started to cry, my husband squeezed my hand and said, "I got this." Even though I was upset, I knew he was right.

CLARE

I was on the phone the day before my delivery, trying to reach a representative who could answer some questions about my benefits during my maternity leave. I was impatient after being on hold for over twenty minutes, which already put me in a foul mood. When he finally took the call and advised me my paperwork was incomplete and he couldn't process my claim or answer any questions, I was so exasperated, I lost it. I started swearing and screaming at him. There was just no more holding it in. In retrospect, that may have actually helped me get ready for delivery. My strong emotions were going to come out at some point, and I certainly entered the hospital much calmer than I would have if I hadn't lost it on the phone with a complete stranger.

It is not uncommon to find something, anything, to hold on to, to feel more grounded during times of higher stress. You might also find yourself potentially lashing out at anyone—even those attempting to help. Keep taking deep breaths to help pace yourself. The lack of control can feel scary and unsettling, but again, your medical team will guide you through what you and your body need to do today.

YOUR ONE RESPONSIBILITY

Your one responsibility (and that of your partner) is to get to the hospital once you're in active labor, or for the scheduled induction or C-section. *That is all.* Your physician and medical team will attend to you from that point forward. While the delivery may not feel straightforward to you, once your body begins labor or your physician begins the C-section, the process itself will carry you through. You just need to first complete your one and only job—showing up.

INPATIENT ADMISSION

Once you arrive at the hospital, whether you present to the triage area, or directly to the labor and delivery floor as a direct admit, you and your partner should ensure that the medical staff is aware of your obstetric history. While your physician and medical team will do their best to communicate well and ensure continuity of care between all providers and across shift changes, there's value in confirming those involved in your care are aware of your circumstances from the first point of contact. That way, no erroneous assumptions are made about who knows what, and the potential for miscommunication is minimized. Care can be that much more individual and sensitive. It can feel awkward to lead with, *"This isn't my first pregnancy; I had a prior loss. I want you to be aware that experience may influence some of my reactions today."* But the alternative of others not knowing and making presumptions about your experience today is arguably worse.

MAEVE

I was uncomfortable and embarrassed to be walking into the hospital, where I knew most women were happy and filled with excitement about meeting their babies. While I was very relieved to have gotten to this point, I also felt sad and kind of sorry for myself that I didn't get to be one of those women who just felt pure joy. I don't blame them, but that single focus doesn't exist for me anymore.

I forced myself to tell the nurse my son died, even though I did not like drawing added attention to myself. She responded with warmth and compassion and said, "I am so, so sorry." Then, she looked me straight in the eyes and said, "We are going to take things one step at a time today, and I'll talk you through it all so you will know what is happening as we go. First, I need to hook you up to the monitors so I can see this baby's activity. We will focus on her today, but if you want to share more with me, I would also love to hear about your son."

My immediate tears were unexpected but were full of relief and gratitude. In that single moment, the nurse freed me from carrying the weight of my past alone, and I realized she kindly and importantly focused my sights on my present.

Some women enter the hospital with a formal birth plan they present to their physician and hospital staff. This plan outlines all their preferences for care and dictates the intended flow from beginning labor through birth. In theory, a great idea. In reality, however, it's very unlikely you will be able to influence or orchestrate every single aspect of this delivery to perfection. Instead, the current status of your medical health and that of your baby's will drive care decisions.

If some preferences or requests can be accommodated, hospital staff are generally willing to oblige, within reason. Communicate with them to explore the realistic possibilities. Be thoughtful and honest about what feels most helpful at each stage, and identify anything that decreases the amount of stress or pressure you feel.

ERIN

We made sure that everyone in the room knew this birth was extremely emotionally charged for us because of our previous loss. We also requested in advance that the baby be given to my husband at delivery to hold first, and not to me. This was hugely helpful for me because it allowed me the space I needed to process the overwhelming mix of emotions that I was sure I would, and did, feel. When I would allow myself to think about the delivery in the weeks before the birth, this was the moment that I focused on. I was terrified of this moment. The baby would be born, immediately placed on my chest, and I would be expected to cry tears of joy and instantly fall in love. But what if all I felt was disappointment because this baby wasn't my daughter? What if I became angry? What if I felt no connection? What if all I wanted was for someone else to be holding this baby because I was emotionally overloaded and needed more time? As soon as we decided to take the pressure off this moment by asking the doctor to hand the baby to my husband, who would give him to me when I was ready, I felt more comfortable. After the baby was born, the doctor gave him to my husband, and I was able to breathe and check in on how I was feeling, instead of being pressured to feel and act a certain way. Much to my surprise, I wanted to hold him shortly after delivery.

Ideally, decisions have long been made about which family members and friends will be invited to the hospital, or present for the actual delivery. Many women continue to opt for extreme privacy, while others may consider additional support for themselves, their partner, and the baby. If you have decided to have anyone present, be specific, clear, and direct with them about your expectations. For example, will that person remain in the family waiting area until after the actual delivery, or be welcome in your labor and delivery room? Take the control you need, especially regarding the things you actually have the power to impact.

ERIN

I've learned that allowing myself the space to feel what I feel for as long as I need to feel it has helped me cope throughout this pregnancy after losing my daughter. In advance of the delivery, my husband and I also let our family and friends know that we would need space and time after the birth to process everything and bond with the new baby and that we would let them know when we were ready for them to meet our son. This may have seemed odd to some, but for me, it was necessary to give myself the best chance to bond with my baby.

THE DELIVERY

As you experience the birth of this baby, you may be overcome with emotions and inevitably evoke your previous pregnancy, independent of whether that experience included a delivery. You will be cognizant of the fact this is not the baby you had once intended to deliver and bring home. That doesn't mean you can't focus on this birth; it means you will see this experience through the eyes of your history—something very unique and individual to each and every woman.

ANDREA

When I was in labor with my son, there was a moment when I must have had a particularly pained look on my face and the nurse said, "I know, this sucks." My response was, "There is a baby coming, there isn't anything about this that sucks." She made a comment about wishing all her patients had such great attitudes, but honestly (and she didn't know this), everything that sucked about my journey was behind me. The physical pain of labor may very well have been one of my greatest joys.

In your head, you may have been playing and replaying the anticipated birth for weeks, if not months, which has heightened the focus and intensity of this event. Your experience is going to be both emotional and physical. Even without a loss history, childbirth itself marks a time of perhaps the greatest vulnerability of a woman's life. That can be a scary situation for women who are already feeling compromised from both the physical demands of pregnancy and the cumulative toll of grief.

ERIN

My contractions came on quickly, so I was pretty much consumed by the pain with little room for feeling anything else until I got the epidural. Once it kicked in, I remember feeling SO much better physically, but that was followed by a huge emotional wave of panic, fear, sadness, and longing for my [deceased] daughter. I had brought her owl blanket (I sleep with it every night) into labor and delivery and held onto it while I cried. (It was important to me to

*have something of hers with me when her brother was born.) At some point, I
calmed down, the doctor broke my water, and our third child was born.*

ALLISON

*The twin pregnancy went normally. The boys grew and I opened up my heart to
them away from fear. And, on the day I was induced, there was no one in the
world who wanted a baby (babies) in her arms more than me.*

*I started contracting at thirty-six weeks, then was admitted for induction at
thirty-eight when my cervix wouldn't dilate. I knew all along it was because of
the D&E [following termination of pregnancy for prenatal diagnosis]. Young physicians' history-taking skills are abysmal, and I didn't feel like talking about my
loss until, finally, a wise nurse practitioner came in and asked. As I told the whole
room of residents in OB and anesthesia, and students galore, that I had had a
D&E and they could refer to my chart, the nurse practitioner moved things along
by releasing the scars from my cervix with her exam. I dilated within thirty minutes. I delivered my first son vaginally, but he was anemic so was whisked away
from me. I calmed my emotions for my second son, but his heart rate bottomed
out, due to a cord compression. The whole room panicked. I was calm. I grabbed
the mask from the anesthesia resident and placed it over my own mouth. I will
never forget that. I was saying, "Put me out, put me out, put me out . . ."*

*When I came out of general anesthesia following the emergency C-section,
there were surgeons around me, and no babies, and no husband. Both boys
had needed NICU care, and my husband went with them. I would like to say
that I didn't have painful flashbacks to the D&E. But I did. There, on the happi-
est day, I was alone again in an operating room with doctors around me, and
no babies and no husband.*

*When we finally held our baby boys all together in the NICU and cried, it
was for all of the reasons new parents do, and so much more. When I look at
the photo we took that day, it reminds me just as much of the journey as the
day itself.*

*The shock of newborn twins definitely came at a time when I didn't have
many emotional "reserves," and I still look back at that newborn time and*

wonder whether some of my behavioral responses to the stress weren't based on the simultaneous battle with grief.

BECKY

The delivery did not bring up any anxieties for me until my water broke and the baby went into distress, and seventeen different people came running into the room to try and resolve the problem. In an instant, I was convinced that this baby would die too. This time seemed like it lasted forever but, in actuality, it was only five minutes. Shortly after the scare, I was ready to push. I used all of my power to push and get the baby out so I would know it would survive. I was so relieved when the baby came out and the doctor asked me if I wanted to hold him. I knew instantly he was fine because the doctor would not have offered him to me if something was wrong. We heard his cry, and the fears that had plagued us for months, immediately disappeared.

At times, you may not be able to be fully present emotionally, which is entirely understandable, finding yourself in and out of memories of the experience of your prior pregnancy or delivery, and this one. Or, the delivery may find you hyperfocused on your physical body and this experience, and completely distracted from your past. If that occurs, know that it takes *nothing* away from your deceased baby, although you may find feelings of guilt begin to emerge for being so focused on this new baby. Each and every experience of delivery is going to be individual and unique.

Work to withhold any judgment and analysis. This is all new, and it is going to take time for you to adjust. Don't rush that—you don't have to say or do anything specific right now. Instead, try to be open to feeling whatever surfaces—grief, pain, relief, excitement, sadness, joy—any and all of it.

This can be a highly emotional and overwhelming time for you, both in good and bad ways. Allow yourself to simply be. Independent of how straightforward childbirth is or is not, what you and your body have just accomplished are truly incredible! Delivery itself is a powerful and tremendous feat, not to mention all you have had to traverse emotionally to get to this point in time.

Be as present as you are able, working to embrace yourself—this moment is a result of all of *your* hard and persistent work. *YOU DID IT!*

THE FIRST FEW POSTPARTUM HOURS AND DAYS IN THE HOSPITAL

As the reality continues to set in that you are now successfully through the experience of pregnancy and birth, your predominant reaction will likely be that of extraordinary relief. You have just successfully given birth to a baby! Your body has yet again shown you all that you are capable of, but you and your body are going to be exhausted. Even though the main event of this pregnancy is behind you, there's still an awful lot happening in the first few hours and days. Everything may feel somewhat surreal as you wrestle with the extreme push-pull between your most recent experience with loss and now new life, and your immediate physical recovery, all while having to wrestle with some immediate decisions.

First Moments with Your Baby

In the first few minutes, hours, and days the two of you are together, take your time and proceed slowly, checking in with yourself with regularity to determine how and what you are feeling. Bonding is highly individual and can occur at various rates and speeds. Don't allow a preconceived idea to dictate or dominate the here and now. Remember, the only expectation at first is for you to meet this baby. You can assess your feelings about him or her over the days and weeks ahead as you begin to gradually explore each other. Do not make comparisons based on what you think your interactions should look like. Instead, just share some space and time together. The goal is to create the opportunity for an emotional attachment to naturally develop. It will happen, but it will be easier for you if you don't force it.

You may find yourself more than a little sensitive to what others think, questioning, *"What will the nurse think if I'm not the one holding my baby?"* That should not be the focus—it matters what *you* think, so when you're tired or need a break, ask your partner or family member to hold the baby. Conversely, you may find yourself overprotective and not wanting anyone else to hold or feed or change the baby. That's okay, but not indefinitely. Remember, your partner is an equal parent to this baby and it's important to allow that emotional attachment to develop as well. Find a balance that works for you both, and let things unfold naturally.

Breastfeeding vs. Bottle Feeding

Decision-making about how and what to feed the baby comes to a head immediately following delivery. Many women plan to breastfeed their babies, believing it to be the best and right thing to do. Sometimes formula is best for the baby if a mother is unable to produce enough milk, the baby doesn't latch, or she simply doesn't want to devote her limited energies and patience to a trial when formula is readily available. Lactation consultants can suggest useful tips and tools, but extraordinary efforts to either produce or maintain a milk supply may have a detrimental impact on the mother's emotional health and well-being.

Women should be impartially counseled that, while they may naturally possess an ideal option through breast milk, the true ideal is to make the decision that works best for each mother and her baby. Bereaved mothers tend to beat themselves up if they don't breastfeed, believing themselves to be bad mothers if they aren't doing what seemingly every other mother on the planet can do spontaneously and naturally. If this is the case for you, try not to prolong this decision or battle unnecessarily. Instead, make the most comfortable and suitable choice for you and your baby. This thoughtful choice will help you to regain some sense of control and confidence about your ability to parent. As any pediatrician will reassure you, babies can grow and thrive whether they are exclusively breastfed, supplemented with formula, or exclusively formula-fed. And in the years to come, no one will know or care which decision you made.

Hormones and Emotions

As soon as you deliver the placenta, your estrogen and progesterone levels begin to drop dramatically and can help prepare your breasts to produce milk. These abruptly lowered levels can also cause feelings of depression, similar to changing hormonal levels that can result in mood swings and irritability before menstruation. Prolactin and oxytocin are two other hormones that will adjust in level after delivery. Prolactin levels will increase after delivery, and every time you pump or breastfeed, creating and storing more milk. Oxytocin is the hormone that helps your breasts actually release the milk. Even though you may feel physically relieved to no longer be pregnant, these rapidly changing hormonal levels can make for an emotional roller coaster.

Feeling down and even tearful is a typical experience for any woman after the dramatic high of childbirth. It is going to take weeks for your hormone levels to balance, and you might experience many emotional ups and downs during this time that may be intensified because of your past.

ERIN

I felt somewhat emotionally numb for the first day after our son was born. It seemed so surreal. I was just at this hospital. I had just given birth to our daughter. She JUST died. Where did this little guy come from? How could he possibly be here? I felt like I was stuck between two worlds.

If, during this time, a wave of emotion hits you, avoid making decisions in the moments you feel most unsteady. Instead, focus on the things that provide comfort and then revisit decisions after you've had some rest, a shower, or a snack. Be kind, gentle, and patient with yourself; this is going to be a process. Your body has just experienced a major trauma, and it's going to take time to begin to heal physically and emotionally.

Given your prior loss, you are at an increased risk for postpartum depression and anxiety, but that does not mean you will automatically experience clinical symptoms. (More on this in Chapter 11, but this topic is important to put on your radar now.) It is standard for physicians to talk with all mothers about postpartum mood and anxiety at the time of their postpartum follow-up appointment, generally four to six weeks after delivery. This period gives the body more time to regulate itself hormonally and to adjust to no longer being pregnant. Ideally, conversations about mental health adjustment are not isolated to a one-time conversation weeks after delivery. You have opportunity to express and share how you are feeling, and for as long as needed, to ensure you have access to the most appropriate level of support and care.

Asking for help isn't always straightforward or easy—especially when you're feeling insecure and vulnerable. And, sometimes, things can be felt to go downhill quickly once home from the hospital when you are not surrounded by trained professionals 24/7 who are helping take care of you and the baby. Consider sharing this with your physician prior to discharge home from the hospital: *"I'm aware of my increased risk for depression and anxiety given my history. Instead of waiting for my postpartum appointment, I'd like some referrals now, just in case."* Then call and schedule your first appointment with this professional *before you leave the hospital,* even if the appointment is booked for several weeks out. A good rule of thumb is to set up a monthly appointment for at least the first six months (and more frequent if needed). Every woman can benefit from additional emotional support postpartum, even if it's determined that longer-term mental health treatment isn't required. It's invaluable to know that if you do need a safety net, it's already in place.

Flashbacks

It is possible you may experience flashbacks to your prior loss in the aftermath of delivery. This may occur not only for you and your partner but sometimes for your family members as well. Your previous pregnancy and delivery can remain active in your mind and stir memories. In time, the flashbacks will dissipate as you integrate both experiences into your history.

You and those close to you may even mistakenly refer to your baby by the name of your deceased baby on more than one occasion. Know that none of this takes anything away from your new baby or the one you lost, nor is your love for either diminished.

MARNEY

I remember just staring at the babies after delivery and wondering how we had gotten here. It was almost like I had PTSD throughout my pregnancy and awoke in this new surreal reality. I was so grateful that I couldn't even express it; instead, I would just cry. One of the babies looked just like our [deceased] daughter, so I had to really work on getting through the flashbacks when I held him.

When he later hit the ten-pound mark [my deceased daughter's birth weight] and was sleeping in my arms is when I had the most trouble. I just had these terrible flashbacks of holding our daughter in the hospital. During these times, I found myself singing "Please don't take my sunshine away" and silently crying as I rocked him. Once he gained some more weight, things got a little easier. I still had trouble holding them when they slept and I still sing that song to them. I probably always will.

TABITHA

I had very mixed emotions upon my son's arrival. I was overjoyed that he was finally here, healthy and safe in my arms, but I remember as the day went on and things calmed down, I couldn't keep it together. We never got past that stage of "moving mom and baby to the recovery room" with our daughter. By the time we moved with her, we had her baptism as quickly as possible and she passed away in my arms shortly after that. So, with my son, it was all just so overwhelming and shocking how NORMAL things were moving along, and it brought back a lot of flashbacks at that point. I remember being in the recovery room crying and hugging our son and my husband because I was simultaneously so happy and relieved but also so very sad that we were robbed of this bonding time with our daughter. And I couldn't help feeling like I had let her down. And, of course, I had many moments of guilty feelings in the hours, weeks, and months after our son was born, and still do sometimes.

Slow down, way down. Give yourself time and set realistic expectations. This delivery has been anticipated for months, and being just hours or a few days beyond delivery will not in itself find you necessarily settled. Pace your-self physically and emotionally as you adjust to no longer being pregnant, to having another baby, and to all the new and emerging roles and responsibil-ities associated with this birth, especially if grief or trauma are reactivated. Take time to let all this newness begin to settle in.

Visits from Hospital Staff

During your hospitalization, you will receive visits from various hospital staff and departments, including some who will ask to take the baby out of your room for a newborn hearing screen, a blood draw, and other routine tests. You can also expect a visit from a representative from the birth certificates department, inquiring about a name for the baby. Although all of these pro-fessionals have long lists of patients to see and limited time to see them, it is always an option to ask them to return later if it's not convenient for you when they drop by. Be polite and respectful, but be direct. Unless something is medically indicated now, most staff are able and willing to return after see-ing other patients.

You can also be very candid with the nursing staff. They will be required to check on you and your vitals with regularity, but you can indicate your prefer-ence as to how much additional privacy or contacts are preferred.

Announcing the Birth and Receiving Visitors

You and your partner exclusively get to decide how and when you announce the news of this birth. Just recognize that as you have been anticipating this day for months, others have too. Family and friends are probably anxious and impatient, awaiting news about you and this baby. You don't owe others im-mediate information but it may be helpful to at least let them know you and the baby are healthy and stable following delivery, even if you plan to keep ad-ditional details private until you have had some rest and more time to adjust. Many couples consider using this opportunity to also send a text or email that reinforces specific wishes: *"It is with great joy we announce the healthy birth of our son. Your continued respect of our privacy is greatly appreciated as we begin to*

get to know him, and also remember the baby we lost before. We'll be in touch soon
with more detail once we are home and settled in."

If you need more time and space before introducing this baby to others, don't feel bad or guilty. Find a sensitive way to express your needs, leaving the door open to receiving visitors in as reasonable a time frame as possible. Once delivery is behind you, you and your partner may feel differently about having family and friends present. If you previously decided against having visitors during or after the birth but suddenly have a change of heart, that's fine—you'll probably make many people happy who are already poised to rush in with pure joy and genuine love. If they visit, however, they may need some direction and guidance to channel their excitement.

Of note, it is a given for family and close friends to want and expect to hold your baby upon first meeting. All women, not just those previously bereaved, can have highly individualized reactions to this desire. Even if you welcome visitors, you may hesitate handing over your newborn to someone else immediately. Ideally, family members should proceed cautiously and take their cues from you and your partner, but this is not always the case. Again, this is a time for you to express your needs and concerns politely but assertively. You can also enlist the help of your nurse who can graciously excuse visitors after a specified amount of time to allow you privacy and much-needed rest.

Visits from a Big Brother or Big Sister

If you have other children at home, consider these suggestions for a more positive introduction when they come to visit:

- **Greet and give your older child your undivided attention at first.** You can do this by asking whether the hospital has a staffed newborn nursery where the baby can be placed temporarily or have another adult wheel the newborn bassinet to and from your room to ensure your arms are first free for your older child. Better to greet that sibling alone and with as much familiarity as possible. This might include wearing your pajamas or robe instead of a hospital gown, or using your usual face or hand cream—things that will help make you and the hospital environment

seem and even smell a bit more comforting. If your older child is a toddler, letting him or her spend some time in the hospital room, playing
with the up/down buttons on the bed, or turning the television on/off,
can be fun. After acclimating to this new space—and you—the baby can
be brought in. This can also be a helpful strategy when exiting the hospital room and even when returning home with the baby: to have someone
else be responsible for your newborn so your arms can be prioritized and
used for your older child first.

- **Prepare for the possibility that leaving your hospital room may not
  be straightforward, especially if your other child is a toddler.** Some
  children struggle with saying good-bye and departing after a visit, not
  wanting to leave you. Try to avoid having the last image your older child
  sees be of you and the baby. Enlist his or her help to return the baby to
  the nursery together, or ask your parent or a friend to watch the baby
  briefly while you have a one-on-one good-bye with your older child.
  Having your partner or parent distract your child with a favorite toy may
  help make the transition from hospital to home much easier. Lots of extra hugs and kisses can go a long way, too, as can a special gift from you to
  your older child as a thoughtful gesture and something tangible to hold
  on the way out of your room.

- **Don't overanalyze whatever happens.** This is a time of newness and
  increased stress for everyone. Be patient and tolerant during this time of
  uncertainty and exploration, giving everyone—including yourself—the
  necessary room to adjust to a new normal.

EARLY DAYS AT HOME

Just as delivery was an emotional experience, returning home can be too. It's
understandable and normal to feel apprehensive leaving the hospital where all
of your needs were being met and help was just a call light away for you and the
baby, who will still require around-the-clock care. Two to three days—even
with good rest—is not much time for your body to recover from the physical
strain of pregnancy, the birth, and the cumulative lack of sleep. It's also not

enough time to even begin processing everything that has just happened from an emotional standpoint. Even once home in familiar settings, emotions are still running high and can be further fueled by adrenalin.

BECKY

Two days later, we were ready to leave the hospital. The nurse walked us out of the hospital and handed us our baby boy, who was named for his [deceased] twin sisters. As soon as we walked out the doors, I started crying hysterically. This was not the moment I thought I would get emotional. Throughout my pregnancy, I never believed we would get to the point where I would be taking a living baby home. I spent the entire pregnancy bracing for the worst, so I never allowed myself to believe that this was real. I had protected myself by not getting attached to the pregnancy or believing that there could be a positive outcome. I cried the whole way home from the hospital out of happiness and despair that this single baby was not my twin girls.

JENNY

We are home! It's great and scary to be home. My husband and I felt like we were total rookie parents last night—we're somehow unprepared, so were kinda scrambling all night. Didn't know where to change her or feed her, didn't have anything to put her in, didn't have my breast pump, no burp cloths, etc. Trying to get a little more organized today! I can't stop crying tears of joy. I can't believe it's all over (and a new crazy is beginning!).

It's entirely okay—expected even—not to have everything figured out at this point, your emotions included. You're likely going to experience a wide and unpredictable range of feeling and, as during delivery, you will do well to avoid all judgment and self-analysis. These first days at home can feel overwhelming, so take the guess work out of it and prioritize the following three main things to establish a solid foundation.

Basic Needs First—the Baby's and Yours!

Even if you come home from the hospital feeling relieved, happy, and excited, the reality soon sets in that this is going to be a lot of work! From newborn care and mountains of laundry, to dishes and household management, the list of needs is endless—even if you don't have another child at home. Focus on meeting the baby's basic needs as well as your own. They are just as important, if not more so, than the baby's. Everything and everyone else can wait, especially during these first few days when you're feeling tired and overwhelmed.

Accept Help from Others

Once home, some women want time away from the baby, preferring to focus on other people or things at first—such as an older child, or even your pet—to tap into a sense of familiarity and comfort. Other women feel overprotective of the baby and unready to allow anyone else to provide care. It can be hard to trust others at first—even your partner or family—but providing full care solo, 24/7, is not realistic or sustainable. Further, this possessiveness prevents your partner and family from developing their own relationships with the baby, and hampers the ability to increase their competence and confidence to relieve you in the future.

Most women fall somewhere in the middle, preferring to spend some time with the baby and some time away. Regardless of where you land, you *can* benefit from help. Do not attempt to do everything alone. It is not sustainable and will exhaust you mentally, emotionally, and physically. There is more than enough work to go around for everyone. Seek out and utilize available and willing help, hiring someone if you need to. You will be able to do much more yourself in time, but not right now.

Once you have help, be specific and direct as to the type of support you need, whether it's household responsibilities or newborn care. Be clear about the tasks to be covered and delegate whatever is less desirable or more challenging for you to undertake, or things you don't have time to handle. Tasks can include laundry, meal prep, or assistance with the baby. If you'd prefer to be alone with your partner, or your partner to be with the baby periodically so you can have quality time with your other child or a friend, speak up. Also be vocal if you don't want to socialize. It's fine to ask a friend to drop off dinner, but not stay for dinner. Being able to lean on others is important and will also ensure you have the possibility of getting some sleep—one of the most essential parts of your physical healing after labor and delivery. Getting proper rest will go miles in helping support your emotional healing.

Regular Self-Care

When you can, take regular breaks away from the baby, and not just to run an errand. Having unstructured time for yourself to do whatever you want—whether it's grabbing a coffee with a friend, taking a hot shower, or going for a fifteen-minute walk—will help you relieve and recenter yourself.

HOME TO STAY—THE FIRST SIX WEEKS

As days turn into weeks, you are still in the aftermath of birth, having just experienced some of the highest highs, but also on the heels of the lowest lows following your prior loss. Your emotions need more time to balance and settle. It is normal and natural to feel unsteady at times, unsure of yourself, and anxious. Physically, your body will continue to heal from the cumulative impact of pregnancy, labor, and delivery, and grow stronger with each passing week. But there's a lot more work sorting out and processing your emotions, some of which may be conflicting, and some of which may not necessarily be resolved in a linear fashion. The roller coaster you were on spanned months and involved some terrifying turns, so you may still feel unsteady even though your feet have touched back down on the ground after pregnancy.

After months of buildup to the crescendo of delivery, it's not uncommon to feel down or even depressed. This is true for *all* women postpartum, but your pregnancy experience wasn't just filled with the anticipation of excitement, it was also filled with the agony of anxiety. You had to pace and brace yourself through each week and it's likely the full reality and impact of all you've been through is only starting to sink in now.

If you haven't already, this is an important time to confirm you are already linked with an individual therapist and that you have your postpartum follow-up appointment scheduled with your physician to continue to assess for postpartum mood changes and anxiety, and receive treatment (including medication) if indicated.

ERIN

I know that babies can die. I watched my daughter. So, I am much more fearful and anxious with my son. At first, sleeping was difficult because I had to constantly check to see if he was breathing. The day after he was born, when we were still in the hospital, he spit up and coughed. This triggered an instant and intense fear. I was terrified and yelled for the nurse, who I'm sure expected to walk in on a much more dire situation than a baby spitting up. I gave him to the nurse until I calmed down, mostly because I knew that if he were to stop breathing, I wouldn't be able to save him. A few nights after he came home, he spit up in his crib and my husband and I both bolted out of bed in terror, ready to call 911 just like we had to do for our daughter. Now that I am on medication and we are feeling more comfortable caring for him, the anxiety with regard to him dying has significantly decreased. But those moments of sheer terror still paralyze me sometimes when I look over and don't immediately see him breathing.

MANAGING PANICKED AND INTRUSIVE THOUGHTS

Some women—even those without a history of loss—may find it difficult to control their worries and fears, as every symptom their baby displays throws them into a state of panic, believing something catastrophic—even death—to be imminent. Anxiety and panic disorders, and post-traumatic stress are real and can make these types of thoughts increase in intensity and frequency. If you find yourself distracted; are unable to quiet, redirect, or regulate these types of thoughts; or if the thoughts negatively impact your ability to perform daily activities or your ability to parent, individual therapy and/or medication is highly recommended. Passing thoughts of worry or concern are different than paralyzing perseverations, obsessions, or compulsions. Cognitive behavioral therapy, in particular, has been proven to be especially effective in these areas, and it can help you feel more comfortable overall as you learn to better understand, and then regulate these thoughts and reactions.

Even if you have help, life at home can still feel like a tough balancing act as the new baby will demand much of the attention and focus of your days and nights. It is normal to still feel frustrated and torn at times, working hard but not always finding a straightforward or comfortable balance between all of your roles and responsibilities.

THE BALANCING ACT CONTINUES

Even with regular help, you may feel there are not enough hours in your days. When this occurs, prioritize the people and things most important and time-sensitive at any given moment. A new normal is being established, and you will need more time to adjust. Communicate honestly and regularly with your partner and discuss reasonable and realistic expectations of each other. He or she is your greatest champion but may be feeling left out, unimportant, dismissed, or even useless as the new baby takes center stage.

Reinforce the importance of your relationship and connection, and find creative ways to maintain regular communication, even if it's a simple sticky note left on the kitchen counter next to drying baby bottles. You are both being pulled in many different directions, and will continue to be. This will leave you feeling torn at times—between this baby and your partner, and between family and friends—that's all to be expected on this stretch of the road.

As a bereaved mother, there is no area this pull feels greater than the felt divided loyalty between this new baby and your deceased baby. However, this is the one area in which you don't have to work hard to communicate, find compromise, or balance time; you can have a deep connection to *both* babies at the same time, and always.

YOUR DECEASED BABY'S PLACE HAS ALREADY BEEN SECURED

Time has shown you that some things change. But time has also shown you that some things are forever. Your love for your deceased baby has not lessened through your experience of subsequent pregnancy, or birth of another baby; that love has and will remain constant. This new baby's presence will continue to prove that your love is not limited or finite. Through this experience, you have confirmed your love is still powerful today and that will continue far into your future. Your deceased baby will forever remain a part of you and you will carry his or her memory, always.

TABITHA

In the weeks and months following our son's arrival, I was okay with the fact that he would be the center of everyone's universe, and there would be little talk about our [deceased] daughter. I expected that and, quite frankly, he deserved it. He was a beautiful blessing to our entire family. I gave him my undivided attention but I knew deep down it wouldn't take away from my bond with my daughter and how often I thought about her. I figured I would rather not set my expectations of people too high because then I would end up hurt and disappointed. So, I tried not to let it bother me when people didn't make many references to her. That way, when someone did, I had that unexpected moment of happiness. Plus, I have always been able to talk about her with my mom and sisters openly, and it's not uncomfortable at all. But with other people, it is sometimes uncomfortable so I almost prefer it to be limited.

I did, and still do, feel guilty sometimes that I think of my daughter less often, but I know that not one day goes by that she is not on my mind. I'm at peace with the fact that although the frequency may have decreased, the depth of her impact on my heart is something that will never change.

Facing this truth will free you to develop your bond with this new baby.

EXPLORING YOUR EMOTIONAL CONNECTION WITH YOUR NEW BABY

The quality and integrity of any human connection are not based on the *quantity* of time shared; they are based on the depth of the attachment. Attachment and bonding are highly individual, not always linear, and should be respected as such. There is no one right way or universal time frame for you to explore this new baby.

BECKY

Family and friends came over to meet our new baby. My family talked about how much they loved him and how they didn't know they could love someone so much. Friends declared their happiness and talked about how cute he was. I found myself not bonding with this baby that I had wanted to bond with so badly. I was not experiencing the same loving feelings that everyone around me kept describing. Instead, I put my focus on making sure that he was fed and then quickly letting someone else hold him. On the inside, I was screaming, "What is wrong with me?!!! How could I not be head-over-heels in love with this baby?!" I was resenting everyone who said they loved him. I also started to get irritated by the outpouring of love we were receiving. We received generous gifts from people who would normally not give us gifts. It was an odd feeling to be getting more gifts because our daughters had died.

As the weeks passed, and with help from a therapist, I started to bond with my son. I am now able to delight in each of his faces, sounds, and movements. I still am struck by sadness when I think about what this would have been like with two babies or how old my daughters would be now. I also find myself wanting to punch people who say your son is here because of your daughters, and this is how it was supposed to be. It is hard for me to think that I have my son because my daughters did not survive. Maybe after more time passes, I will be able to see things that way but for now, I am happy with my son and continue to miss my daughters.

TABITHA

I can honestly say I never had an issue bonding with my son. If anything, I bonded with him easily because I looked at him and saw that he was a part of my husband, his [deceased] sister, and myself all in one. And I was going to hold on to him for dear life and cherish every moment we had. And, in all honesty, I believe he is a gift from his sister because, as harsh as it sounds, he would most likely not be here had she not passed away.

I often look at him and wish I had these same experiences with my daughter but it never prevents me from loving and enjoying this time with him. He is his own person and I can separate my emotions about his sister (whether it be happy, angry, sad, guilty) from what I feel for him during various events or circumstances. I often have a feeling of longing to see, hear, and feel these things with my daughter, too, but I don't let that interfere with how I treat my son.

Remember, the expectation was *not* to fall in love with the baby upon first sight at delivery; the expectation was simply to *meet* him or her. Now, the task is to continue to get to know this baby, and that may occur gradually and at your own pace. Relationships take time to build, and even if you had positive and strong feelings of attachment at the time of delivery, there will be times in the future when you feel detached, disconnected, and even upset and angry with this child. That is part of parenthood. Mixed, conflicting, and rapidly changing feelings will continue to surface well beyond delivery through the toddler years, the teen years, and into adulthood.

Some women don't experience neutral or negative feelings for some time. Other women experience them before feeling positive attachment and a bond. There is no right or wrong. Both are possible. This is not something unique to the delivery of a subsequent baby after a loss, but true for all parents. Understanding this reality can be liberating and preferable to caving in to the unnecessary pressure of needing to feel a certain way. Any concerns you have about the possibility of under- or overattachment can best be explored in individual therapy where you can better process your feelings about this new baby, and receive helpful guidance.

Time and patience are the greatest gifts you can give yourself in the early postpartum period. Feelings and reactions will continue to be unpredictable for some time. Some women sail through delivery seamlessly only to fall apart after, whereas some fall apart before or during but stand strong after. It remains a very individual experience. What you should focus on is that you already took the greatest fall after losing your pregnancy or baby, but you got back up and on the track toward parenthood. You will have setbacks as a parent, and there will be many times when your confidence will wane. But that will not stop or change the integrity of your commitments. You've long proven you are a dedicated and loving parent.

With each passing day, again, your body is growing stronger physically and your experience with this baby is becoming more and more real. You are already gaining in competence and confidence with ever-growing experience in caring for and parenting this baby. As days become weeks, you're realizing this is where you can take more control and decide what you will set down, and what you will continue to carry. You can continue to uphold your relationship with your partner and others you love and who love you. You will find ways to carry the memory of your deceased baby along with your deepening relationship with this new baby. You are also beginning to realize that following your experience of past trauma, you can now carry the triumph of birth after death, and the true triumph of *you*.

JACKIE

I love the feeling of an empty belly while I lie on my back in bed. It means I did it—I gave birth to a healthy baby who is sleeping peacefully beside me (for the moment). Her existence was far from certain. In fact, during my nearly three years of fertility treatments, there were many possible exits I could have taken. The odds were very much against us. And in the early days after her birth, I went through a period of doubt—she doesn't look like me because we used an egg donor, and I will one day have to explain this to her. Finally, though, my mind settled upon the very strong fact that I MADE HER—more than most mothers can claim to have made their children since it took so many years of soul-searching determination and seemingly insurmountable obstacles. She exists because of me and my love—this is what I will tell her.

﹛ 11 ﹜

The First Year

WEEKS AFTER DELIVERY, YOU MAY still find great comfort in simply having your body back to yourself. Even if you are frustrated that the pregnancy weight is not coming off as quickly as you want, your physical body is growing stronger with each passing week. On some level, variations on this now familiar tug of war between progress and frustration will continue indefinitely. Still, the fluctuations in this next year won't be anywhere near as dramatic as they have been in the past. You're learning that even with new challenges, you're gaining more and more traction by also experiencing some new successes. Those successes will only continue to grow in number (as some of the prior challenges slip away). You will ride out the normal waves of new parenthood better if you continue to prioritize yourself and work to strengthen your foundation, both physical and emotional. This will help ensure you remain grounded and open to receiving the many joys and gifts that lie ahead for you as a woman, and especially as a mother.

THE SIX-WEEK APPOINTMENT: CONFIRMING PHYSICAL HEALING AND MENTAL HEALTH CHECK-IN

If you delivered vaginally, you will be counseled to schedule your postpartum appointment with your physician approximately six weeks after delivery. In the case of a C-section, most physicians advise for a return OB appointment two weeks after delivery to allow for a preliminary incision check and then again at the six-week mark.

This six-week appointment primarily focuses on a physical examination to ensure your body is recovering well. It also includes a brief conversation about contraception and adjustment to life with a newborn at home (including any breast- or formula-feeding challenges). In some states—New Jersey, Illinois, and West Virginia—a mandatory screen for depression, such as the Edinburgh Postnatal Depression Scale (EPDS) or the Patient Health Questionnaire-9 (PHQ-9), is required. Both these tools involve a series of ten multiple-choice questions that cover the scope of your feelings and functioning over the past one to two weeks.

Although the content of that discussion is essential, the entire standard postpartum follow-up appointment is generally fifteen to twenty minutes in length, meaning that the topics can only be addressed superficially despite the best of provider intentions. Unfortunately, this small window leaves little time to also explore the additional and genuine challenges related to a bereaved woman's prior loss and the impact on her present. Even if providers can engage in conversations of greater depth, it can be challenging to differentiate signs and symptoms of postpartum depression as they may, at first, look identical to reactivated grief. It's easy to see how a new mother could slip through the cracks at a time when she could most benefit from a strong mental and emotional safety net.

Fortunately, awareness has grown and the conversation about emotional/ mental health and healing is becoming more consistently initiated. Further, the American College of Obstetricians and Gynecologists (ACOG) is currently working to shift from a single six-week postpartum visit to a process that allows for more individualized follow-up. This is a significant step in the right direction since, for many women, this appointment is generally the last contact with a physician until the time of her recommended annual exam, one full year later!

As change continues to take place within the medical system to support a smoother transition out of postpartum care, you must take charge of your health and remain committed to efforts that support continued and longer-term healing. That includes getting good sleep, rest, nutrition and hydration, regular exercise once you're cleared to resume activity, and making other healthy lifestyle choices that will support your overall physical and mental health and healing efforts.

POSTPARTUM MOOD AND ANXIETY

According to the Centers for Disease Control (CDC), 1 in 10 women experience depression, and 1 in 9 women, or 11 percent who give birth in the United States, experience symptoms of postpartum depression.[1] (Those numbers are even higher, as the CDC reports only on women with live births.)

As noted in Chapter 1 (but necessary to repeat here), key symptoms of clinical depression, as outlined by the American Psychiatric Association,[2] include at least five of the following that are experienced for most of the day, nearly every day (by self-evaluation or others' observations), and over a two-week period:

- Depressed mood
- Markedly diminished interest or pleasure in all or almost all activities
- Significant weight change (loss or gain) or appetite disturbance
- Insomnia or hypersomnia
- Psychomotor agitation or retardation
- Fatigue or loss of energy
- Feelings of worthlessness, or excessive or inappropriate guilt
- Diminished ability to think or concentrate; indecisiveness
- Recurrent thoughts of death, suicidal ideation

The Centers for Disease Control[3] suggests symptoms of postpartum depression are similar to symptoms of clinical depression, but may also include:

- Increased tearfulness
- Anger
- Withdrawal from loved ones
- Feeling numb or disconnected from the baby

- Worry about hurting the baby
- Guilt about not being a good mother or doubting the ability to care for the baby

Further, the CDC[4] identifies additional risk factors that place some women at an even higher risk for depression:
- Stressful life events
- Low social support
- Previous history of depression
- Family history of depression
- Difficulty getting pregnant
- Being a mother to multiples (for example, twins, triplets)
- Being a teen mother
- Preterm labor and delivery (before 37 weeks' gestation)
- Pregnancy and birth complications
- Having a baby who required hospitalization

The Mayo Clinic[5] of Rochester, Minnesota, adds these considerations and risks:
- The baby has health problems or other special needs.
- There are breastfeeding difficulties.
- There are relationship difficulties with a woman's partner.
- There are financial issues.
- The pregnancy was unplanned or unwanted.

Regardless of environmental stress and other potential influencing factors listed here, the experience of loss alone exacerbates the natural risk for mood symptoms at times of hormonal changes, such as in the first few weeks following delivery.

According to Postpartum Support International,[6] approximately 10 percent of women postpartum will develop anxiety. Risk factors include a personal or family history of anxiety, previous perinatal depression, or thyroid imbalance. Symptoms may include:

- Constant worry
- Feeling that something bad is going to happen
- Racing thoughts
- Disturbances of sleep and appetite
- Inability to sit still
- Physical symptoms, such as dizziness, hot flashes, and nausea

All women postpartum, but especially those with a loss history, can benefit from education about mental health during this time of extraordinary change and adjustment. Many may also gain from continued counseling by licensed professionals who are well trained to provide vital emotional and psychological support, and prescribe and monitor medication if needed. Postpartum depression and anxiety are treatable, but they must first be identified.

ERIN

I decided to go back on an antidepressant after our second son was born so that I could give myself the best chance to bond with him, and care for him, myself, and my family. He is one now, and I've come off the antidepressants. Now that I'm off the medication, I'm feeling a much larger emotional range and am grieving my daughter more intensely than I had been this past year. While part of me feels guilty for effectively pausing the intense emotions that go along with grieving for my daughter, I do still think it was a good decision to stay on it over the last year. Without it, I'm not sure that I would have been able to enjoy my second son or get to a point where I can have and manage my intense emotions.

By taking your mental health just as seriously as your physical health, and remaining committed to prioritizing it long after your six-week postpartum appointment through your continuing work with an individual therapist, you will move yourself in the direction of improved health and healing. Your progress will be more straightforward and your pace arguably faster with professional help and support versus trying to navigate all on your own.

COMMON EMOTIONAL AND MENTAL HEALTH
CHALLENGES FOR ALL WOMEN POSTPARTUM

Even without a clinical mood or anxiety disorder, the professional and community support you've identified can help you adjust to all your new roles and responsibilities, including these four main challenges that are normal for any woman during the first year, not just those with a history of loss:

1. Building competence and confidence
2. Reentering and reacclimating to the world at large
3. Managing feelings of guilt
4. Establishing balance

Your loss history, however, can add an additional challenge, but before you start to feel anxious, disbelieving you have what it will take, *stop*! Look how far you've already come. Look at who and what you have created. You've got this. Keep taking one step at a time and remember you don't have to figure it all out at once or alone. Enlisting the help of professionals is not a sign of weakness; it can help ensure the foundation you are working so hard to create is sturdy enough to endure.

Building Competence and Confidence

Confidence—in oneself and one's maternal capacity—is something most women, and especially those bereaved, struggle with postpartum. Many women don't like how they look physically, especially if they're not back to prepregnancy weight as quickly as they wish. (You are the one who cares most about this; other people care about how you are feeling and doing emotionally. Follow their lead here. Being healthy is always going to be more important than being a certain size.)

Most women are not getting enough uninterrupted sleep, so they are operating at a regular deficit. There is an enormous amount of new information to learn and absorb, and it can take time for you to feel that motherhood is more intuitive, natural, and automatic. Although diaper changing is becoming more routine, swaddling, even with practice, isn't always straight-forward unless you're a professional postpartum nurse. The baby's feeding and sleep schedules are two areas that can also create considerable and ongoing stress. These can leave you feeling helpless, panicked, and lost when the baby doesn't eat as much as expected, spits much of it back up, and is all over the map in terms of falling asleep and waking up.

Partners usually return to work quickly, but even with hired help, you might feel alone and insecure, and compare yourself to other mothers you see who are independent, happy, or juggling more than one child (and the family dog) with ease. Even if you were able to stave off judgment during your labor and delivery, you might be wondering how you now measure up to others. This adds nothing positive, only unnecessary stress and pressure.

When you are out with your baby and tempted to compare yourself to another mother and child, remember, you are comparing yourself to another's *exterior presentation*. Just because she can get her baby in and out of the car seat and secured into the stroller doesn't mean it was so easy the week before. And, if she looks freshly showered, consider that it may have been her first in two days!

Strive to be kinder and more patient with yourself. The expectation during the entire first year of this baby's life is that new learning continues, not to establish yourself as an expert. Babies change a LOT during the first year and just when you feel you may have achieved mastery of something (such as your baby's nap schedule), the baby will change again (such as dropping a nap altogether), throwing a wrench into the routine you thought you had just established.

This can be frustrating for any parent, but because of your loss history, the lack of predictability and control, and subsequent lack of confidence may feel especially unsettling. You may find yourself an overprotective parent, worrying that every cry, every response, or lack thereof, is a sign that something is wrong with your baby, kicking up fears of doom. You may not trust or allow others, including your partner or family members, to provide primary care to this baby, only barely trusting yourself. This may create tension, leaving your partner feeling less than, and left out. Best advice? Slow down. Way down. Take things one day at a time, or even five minutes at a time, as needed. And remember, you don't have to—and shouldn't—go it alone.

You have a support team—your partner, your pediatrician, professionals, and trusted others—and you can and should lean on and communicate regularly with them for additional encouragement, guidance, tips, tricks, and help finding answers to all your many questions. Over time, you will learn to read your baby's cues and figure out the things that work and the things that don't. Don't worry about what's recommended in some baby book; the advice may or may not work for your baby. You will grow in knowledge and experience as you get to know your baby and become more acclimated as a mother. Rest assured, time and continued practice will afford you more competence and confidence. Instead of fixating on your frustrations over everything you don't yet know or understand, celebrate all you *have* learned and are learning during the first year. This is all still very new, so keep doing what you're doing because it gets better, *much* better.

Reentering and Reacclimating to the World at Large

Insecurity about your parenting abilities, your social anxieties (historic, or exacerbated following your loss), and even a fear of germs may initially be barriers to you regularly interacting with others or leaving home with your baby. You may also feel awkward attempting to make new friends at this point—even with other new moms—wanting to avoid uncomfortable and potentially triggering comments or conversations that generalize the experience of new parenthood before you've had the opportunity to increase your confidence, much less affirm your new maternal identity.

Providing care for your baby even at home can feel overwhelming, much more so doing this out in a more public setting. But if you remain homebound, you may battle feelings of increasing loneliness and isolation. There are far greater benefits to you and your baby in acknowledging your discomforts and irrational fears instead of hiding from them, allowing them to block your access to the world at large, or worse, multiply. The professional network you've secured can also support you in taking gradual steps out and back into your community.

Following your loss, you were acutely aware of how alone you felt in comparison to the rest of the very fertile world. You desperately longed to be a part of that world, full of life and color and flavor. Well, that rich and vibrant world is still there, but it's up to you to rejoin it. Because you have felt excluded and somehow different for so long, reentry will take some time. And, understandably, the task can feel harder with a baby in tow.

Consider this example: If a pilot recognizes she or he is ninety degrees off course for an intended destination, and makes a sharp right-angle turn to correct, this maneuver would create considerable upset and turbulence for everyone on board the aircraft. However, the pilot can still nail the landing by making a few subtle calibrations over a short period of time to steer the plane back on course, and ensure a smoother ride for all.

The message here is you don't need to become the most social person overnight, but it is healthy to reestablish some connections with the world at large. Keep your sights focused on your longer-term destination and make careful adjustments as needed to keep yourself on course. Here are some specific strategies for getting you and your baby out of the house and back into the world in a way that may feel more comfortable, and doable.

What You Can Do:
- **Start small.** If you anticipate feeling self-conscious, embarrassed, or trapped if the baby is fussy in a public setting, such as a restaurant, frequent less crowded venues. For example, take your baby for a short walk around your neighborhood or for a car ride, where it is just the two of you.
- **Be prepared.** Always carry extra diapers, wipes, and a change of clothes for your baby. Or you'll learn the hard way.
- **Don't go it alone at first.** Sometimes venturing into new territory can feel less daunting when you're not alone. Bring along your partner or a trusted friend for company. A bonus is that you can also enlist that

person to help carry the diaper bag. This can leave your hands free to tend to your baby.

- **Consider strategic destinations.** You will get in and out of a café or fast-food eatery faster than a sit-down restaurant for a meal, even if that restaurant is family-friendly. Seek out places in which you feel most comfortable and where your baby won't be at all out of place, even welcomed.

- **Learn to tolerate well-intentioned (but unsolicited) advice with grace.** Everyone has ideas about how babies should be cared for and raised, whether they've had experience parenting or not. When someone shares their believed wisdom, it does not mean you're doing something wrong, or even that their advice is right! Recognize you can't control the influx of well-intentioned suggestions. You can smile and accept these recommendations, even if you never end up using them. Or you may also decide to consider trying something new, especially if what you're doing doesn't seem to be working.

- **Try to roll with it.** Just as others want to share advice, they'll also have plenty of questions, including, *"Is this your first?"* and *"How many children do you have?"* People are going to be curious and interested. After all, you have to admit, your baby is pretty cute. It's almost impossible to avoid this common line of questioning when you're out, and it can stir up sensitivities given your past. There are no right or wrong answers, and depending on a million different variables, your answers may not always be the same. There is nothing wrong with sharing information about your past. And there is nothing wrong with keeping it to yourself. If you don't mention your deceased baby, you are not minimizing or forgetting him or her. You are merely choosing to keep very personal information private.

AMANDA

We have a long history. We started with the worst possible tragedy a parent can experience [full-term death of our daughter] and eventually ended up with four healthy boys ... the last were a spontaneous twin pregnancy. It's an amazing and powerful ending to our journey of building a family. But I still get layers of questions. The most common ones now when people see me with four boys are, "Oh, are you gonna try for a girl now?" and "Oh my God, FOUR BOYS?!" Sometimes I have the strength to say, "Our daughter died before they were all born. So, yes, we're done." But other times, I just smile (while in my mind, I say her name).

The questions become a part of your life. I was at Costco with all four boys one afternoon, running errands. Another shopper stopped us and made some acknowledgment about me having four kids and that they are all boys. It was one of those moments when I felt weak and not willing to share, so I chose the smile and nod approach and continued to keep walking. As I was walking away, she said out loud, "No girls? Man, you've been robbed!" It was like a dagger in my back. I stopped for a brief second as I lost my breath and held back tears, and kept moving. I know she didn't intentionally mean to hurt me. But it just goes to show you never know what another stranger's story is, so be kind.

ALLY

I was out with my baby, and someone said, "Your baby is just adorable! How many children do you have?" Without missing a beat or caring whether or not I would make someone uncomfortable, I said, "I have two. I lost my daughter, and then we went on to have this little boy. Thank you for asking; I appreciate being able to talk about them both." The woman looked at me with tears in her eyes and replied, "I am so sorry." And I said, "Thank you. But I'm not. After all that's happened, I'm still so grateful I had both."

So, then, this woman gently touched my arm and said, "I lost a baby, too. Years ago. But I was too scared to try again and never did. I know you don't know me, but I'm so glad you made a different choice." This woman was a complete stranger, but we ended up having a real and meaningful conversation. It doesn't always happen this way when I speak up, but I'm always uplifted when it does.

Work to establish a realistic expectation. There will be some inevitable falls and fails as you reenter and reacclimate with the rest of the world. Over time, by gradually resuming some regular interaction with others and the world at large, your child will learn to become comfortable and sociable around others, and understand that he/she is not your exclusive and singular focus—something vital for you both. And, you will expand this child's horizons by introducing him or her to the community and larger world and through the example you set. You will either teach him your anxieties and limits, or you will teach him all about infinite possibilities and the importance of human connections and relationships. This is a great gift you can give as a parent, and the opportunity and choice are yours. More experience will build more confidence and, eventually, more comfort. Both these things will serve as a bridge into the world at large, which is good for both you and your baby on many levels. So, don't wait on this; get out there and get going!

Managing Feelings of Guilt

As your confidence, competence, and ability to get out more regularly with your baby all grow, it should also become more straightforward to get out to do things for yourself. That may be a return to work, it may be a return to the gym. However, guilt has a way of creeping in and leaves many mothers with bad and negative feelings over having "left" their baby at home, or for not being always present or not wanting to be present, and even not wanting to be a mom sometimes. Let's face it; motherhood is tough and it's demanding, and these types of thoughts are a reflection of those challenges *not* your attachment and commitment to your baby. You may start to think you're not a very good mother because you're not doing more, or not doing enough. Stop right there. Giving time and attention to other responsibilities or priorities (for example, your own physical or emotional health and well-being) are both important and good. Don't look at it as taking away anything from your baby; instead, frame it as honoring and upholding commitments, or as giving to yourself (which in turn will give you more to give back to your baby). These are *not* selfish acts; they are critical acts of self-care and will help support the multidimensional woman you are at your core.

Additionally, you may also find you have some feelings of guilt as your attachment and connection grow beyond what you had experienced in your previous pregnancy or with your deceased baby, or as you continue to grow stronger and experience more joy. This can feel uncomfortable and difficult to reconcile. Remember that each pregnancy and each baby is unique and special, and you will always have different associations with each. The bonds will not be identical, nor should you try to make them feel that way. What is important is that both bonds are everlasting and one takes nothing away from the other.

MARNEY

I have struggled with living with the loss and not feeling guilty about it, questioning all the "what ifs." I look at my twins and tear up, knowing that they may not have been here if things had gone as initially planned. That makes me feel guilty, too, but I want women to know that they can survive. I want to tell other women the things that I didn't hear from someone who had been through it before. I have learned to be more grateful and appreciative of what I have. I have also learned that the support of others is nothing to take lightly. Don't get me wrong, I still have moments of complete craziness where I am so stressed out and tired and agitated, and that also causes guilt. But I do find I check myself a little more often and remind myself that I/we have lived through one of the worst nightmares that parents could have. We will live, love, and survive through this.

Establishing Balance

Over the course of the first year (and beyond), there are going to be times the world feels upside down and out of your control, but you are coming to realize that you can ride those waves and emerge on the other side. Instead of fighting moments or people outside your immediate control, you've found ways to tolerate some discontent and discomfort until you can find calmer space and a clearer head. Part of the work during this first year is finding ways to keep bringing yourself back to center.

With Time

Even if you have full-time help, this new baby is going to command a lot of your time and attention. It is critical for you to prioritize and hone your time management skills to ensure you not only have quality time with this baby, but also with your partner, other children, and your family and friends. This also includes planning regular unstructured downtime for *yourself* to do whatever you wish, even if it's just for an hour. But how is it possible to fit all this into a busy day?

If you are working full-time, you may feel even more pressure (or may want) to spend all of your evening and weekend time with your baby and partner, and/or guilty if you don't. Just remember, the hours and days pass quickly and before you know it, it's Sunday night. So, in addition to sharing meaningful (and fun) time together with your partner and family, factor in time just for you.

One way to get some "me time" is by tag-teaming. You can ask your partner to watch the baby while you head to the gym. Upon your return, switch roles, with you assuming the primary caregiver role. When doable, tag-teaming allows you and your partner windows of time to do things for yourselves that is equitable. You'll both have peace of mind knowing that your baby is well cared for while you're gone too.

Try to balance your time to ensure you have that quality family time, yet also make time for exercise, to meet a friend for coffee, or finally clean out that closet you've been meaning to tackle. No one has enough hours in their days so it's important to use the ones you do have wisely and creatively. Yes, this baby is a huge priority, but make sure you keep others closest to you—and yourself— at the top of the list as well. Even if you are a full-time stay-at-home mom, you are a multidimensional woman! Not only do you serve yourself well by supporting your other interests and passions (all while chipping away at your to-do list), but you also demonstrate independence and self-care for your child.

In Relationships

In many ways, this baby took center stage after delivery, but if he or she becomes your exclusive focus, other areas of your life—including all your relationships—will become imbalanced. Intentionally create one-on-one time with your other children, even if it's for fifteen to thirty minutes of quality interaction at a time. Plan time to check in and connect with your partner, too. If you don't have childcare at night or are too tired to head out for dinner or a date night, consider asking someone to watch your baby during the day so you can meet up for an occasional quick lunch. A lunch or evening out with girlfriends is another way to have fun and stay connected with your friends. It's obvious that your relationships with your partner, family, and friends will look different now that you have a baby at home, but the best way to maintain those relationships is by nurturing them. You'll find a new rhythm to these meaningful connections but it will involve prioritizing, practice, and persistence.

Inside Your Head

Even after you establish a new overall sense of life balance with your time and within your relationships, there's much to be gained by paying attention to your mental and emotional health. This doesn't happen automatically; balancing your mind must be intentional. You will need to weed out your insecurities and worries so you don't get snagged or stuck. Continue to make room for growing competence, confidence, and your greatest hopes. You already have the tools and can use them well; you just need to *remember* to use them. This work will be ongoing as new challenges and concerns emerge throughout your life as both a parent and an individual. The push-pull you'll feel is natural. Life is always dynamic, both in positive and negative ways. Don't fight it; simply recognize and respect that dual reality.

There will always be some distinction between your life before your loss and your life after. However, the emphasis here is that there *is* an "after." This life is not what you had once expected, but you are proving over and over again that there is indeed life after loss—literally with this new baby, and figuratively, with your emerging identity you are continuing work to affirm. True balance and strong and sound emotional health are only found and then maintained when you are able to integrate your past (through acceptance of what has occurred and remains a part of you), your present, and your emerging future.

⸙ 12 ⸙

The Rebirth of You

As the months continue to pass and mark a full year, you will come to realize that you have built your foundation well, and from it, can see your joys deepening and your successes exponentially increasing. You will have seen your baby smile for the first time, raise his head, grasp an object, roll over, laugh, and sit up. You will have witnessed her crawl, clap, pull herself up to stand, utter her first words, and likely take her first steps. Parenthood is stressful, and at times draining, but the accomplishments and growth are tremendous. And, those accomplishments are in large part, because of you and your hard work as a mother to this baby.

Family and friends will also celebrate and focus on these milestones, which are both appropriate and healthy. However, they don't always recognize that the arrival of a new baby is not simply a "reset" after a loss. Well-meaning comments, such as *"At last, you can be happy again!"* or *"You finally got everything you wanted!"* can minimize your experience and dismiss the complex nature of everything you have lived through.

⸙ **ANDREA**

My mom said, "It turned out all right in the end." Without diminishing the utter joy and beauty of my children, the path that led to them can never be justified.

That is not easy for the rest of the world to understand. I feel pretty strongly that the journey and the destination are two of the most exclusive events imaginable. I am eternally grateful for my children. But the endless joy that they bring does not in any way diminish how downright shitty many years of my reproductive life were. The tragedy stands on its own. It always will.

The tragedy will stand and remain an undeniable part of your past. It doesn't, however, have to define you, and it certainly hasn't defeated you. For a long time, your identity was primarily influenced by your grief and loss, overwhelming and all-consuming at various points. But you did not get stuck in it or buried beneath it. You dealt with it head on, eyes wide open, and over time, learned to recognize that taking steps forward did *not* mean taking steps away from your deceased baby. You found ways to not only survive through your grief, but also succeed in bearing new life.

You have emerged and are now solidly on the other side. In some ways, you're worse off because of your past, but there are some ways you are different, even better. To be clear, you're not better out of loss. You're better because you've found ways to confront your fears and not allowed them to paralyze you—and perhaps overcome some of them. You're better because you have confirmed the things and people most important in this world and no longer compromise your time or burden yourself with things and people that are not. You're better because your baby existed, touched you deeply, and is someone you will always hold close. You are better because you have *finally* started to believe in yourself, your body, and your future again. And, over this first year (and as you will see in all the years upcoming), you're better because you've truly started living again, and that is perhaps one of the best ways you can honor your past, and your baby.

NAMI

I sat in the synagogue next to my husband on the first day of Rosh Hashanah and listened to the rabbi's sermon . . . as an elderly lady in the row behind us

leaned over and said simply to me "You and your husband make beautiful chil-
dren. I hope you know how truly blessed you are."

Recurrent pregnancy loss is devastating. It is physically and emotionally
painful, crippling, and often paralyzing. It is frightening, destructive, and lonely.
Yet, despite all the terrible realities of living through a pregnancy after multiple
prior losses, I am also grateful to know how it feels to be on the other side of it.
Women going through recurrent pregnancy loss need to know that they are not
alone. They also need to have hope. For my husband and I, while the physical
and emotional toll of the many rounds of IVF and multiple pregnancy losses
seemed, in the moment, to be insurmountable, thankfully, our desire and resolve
to expand our family was even stronger. And that is why two weeks ago on Rosh
Hashanah, as we sat in the synagogue with our beautiful children and wished
those around us a happy, healthy, and sweet new year, I could say confidently
to the elderly woman in the row behind us that we do in fact know how truly
blessed we are. I know I'm stronger and more resilient than I otherwise would
be, and that is the trait that I hope, most of all, I am able to teach my children.

Your work now is not only focusing on supporting this baby's continued
growth and development, but also affirming your own as a strong and increasingly competent and confident woman and mother.

The affirmation of your new identity postloss, and also postdelivery, is as
much about self-acceptance as it is about self-improvement, both of which can
be very powerful. Your interests, passions, and multidimensional nature are
all still there, waiting and wanting to be rediscovered, watered, and grown in
new and different ways. You now have the power to find peace with the past,
embrace the present, and completely open yourself up to everything the future has to offer.

ERIN

Before our son's birth, I worried that he would steal some of the space in my
heart reserved for our [deceased] daughter. My fear caused me to be somewhat

emotionally guarded with him at first. But I soon realized that he wasn't a threat. Not only did he allow my heart to grow, but he also undeadened it in many ways. He made me realize that there was an untouchable and unique place in my heart for each of my children. Like our oldest son, this new baby boy is his own person with his own place in our family who will carry his sister with him in his own way. Even though he never got to meet her, I feel like they will always have a special connection.

I am not the same person I was before my daughter died. I have become a more authentic and empathetic person who looks at the world from a different perspective. In the rebuilding of myself after her death, values shifted, and old fears were shed. I left my career, moved to a new city, and went back to school to pursue a degree in a profession that allows me to connect with and empower others. Without my daughter, I would not be the person I am today. I am grateful to my daughter for continuing to teach me how to be a better human. ∽

If you haven't already, as you reflect on and remember your past, you will see a major transformation occur. The deep hollow created by your pain and sadness is being replenished over time by a rush of increased depths of patience, empathy, gratitude, and love. That includes the love you experienced for your deceased baby, the deepened love you feel for this new child, plus the new and deepening appreciation and love for who you have become. You're more confident, surer of yourself, more honest, and much more real. No matter what life has thrown your way, you have proven you cannot be kept down.

JANE

I threw away all of my syringes, old vials of medication, alcohol swabs, and written instructions that were the only lingering evidence of my efforts to get to today. The bruises on my belly and hips from the daily hormonal injections are long gone, and those areas now sport stretch marks that I don't like, but that remind me of the strength and amazing resilience of my body. It felt wonderful to finally get rid of all of that and say, "I made it to the other side; I'm

DONE!" No more fighting—against time, with doctors, with the insurance company, with my husband, with myself. But I was surprised to also feel somewhat strange; in a way, empty. Maybe because that used to be my entire world. My days revolved around my fertility treatments for years. I had canceled trips and plans with friends and family, called in sick to work to accommodate egg retrievals, transfers, and then surgical procedures when it initially worked for only a little while, and then until it finally worked to the end. It felt odd to just throw that all into the trash.

But I soon realized the emptiness I felt inside wasn't bad. It was just unfamiliar.

The place that had been filled with depression, anxiety, and uncertainty was now being opened up for other things to take their places. No one will ever take the place of my son, but I've found a way to make room for things like this new baby and her smile and her laugh. And, my own smile and laugh. My God, I've missed that.

AMY

Pregnancy loss has made me a more "in the moment" person. I learned that I need to enjoy the now and not worry so much about planning and trying to control the future. The loss of control has forced me to be more flexible and more forgiving, both of myself and others. Although I am far from perfect, I have a level of patience with my kids that I would not have had without my losses. When I'm having a hard day or have heard "MAMA, I need this . . . ." for the millionth time, I remember how lucky I am to be able to hear them and be needed.

Metamorphosis

Each waking
again
realizing
your death
Paralyzed by pain

Layers upon layers
of grief
How can this be my life?

Endless tears
Strangers making way
sensing our loss
Waves of grief our wake
palpable to passersby
My emotions are an abyss
Is my life now a fossil?

One moment
the sun breaks through
I will not throw myself
into your grave
I know nothing else
not one thing else
It is the way forward
It is enough
Is my life a cocoon sheltering me for the future?

Other humans have survived loss
Hope lies in their stories
Others are strong and brave
and survive
Maybe they could be me,
If I read their stories into my life

Rising from your ashes
My own ashes
evidence of the pyre of my life

My love for you the seed which now fuels me
Maybe instead of a butterfly
I am a phoenix.

   —BRITTANY

Life is admittedly very different than you, or any bereaved woman, ever expected it would be. *But there is still life.* And . . . there is *rebirth*, even after
death. In Greek mythology, the phoenix is a legendary and majestic bird that
possesses the incredible capacity to be cyclically renewed or reborn, able to
live for five hundred years before rising triumphantly from death, reborn to
live again. Over and over again, new life can and does emerge. You've experienced that, and you now not only see it, you've come to believe it . . . even if it
feels as if it took five hundred years to realize.

Epilogue
Never Forgotten

TO RECOGNIZE AND REMEMBER BEREAVED parents and their babies, October was designated as National Pregnancy and Infant Loss Awareness Month on October 25, 1988, by then president Ronald Reagan. Although the entire month is being increasingly observed, the designated day of commemoration is October 15. On this day, people light a candle at seven p.m. that results in a continuous wave of light across time zones and around the world. This is an excellent time of year to annually reflect and act in meaningful ways, whether private and informal, or more public and ceremonial.

Of course, there will be other days or moments in which you wish to remember. Only you can determine what feels most comfortable and significant to you, and that may change over time. Talk with your partner to discuss your ideas, and consider the following four ways to recognize and honor your deceased baby, your past, and yourself.

Reflect

There will be moments throughout your life when you find yourself unexpectedly brought back to a point or time in the past. Although some of the memories you access can be painful, reflecting on them can be intentional and purposeful, and even provide comfort.

233

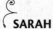

SARAH

Every year on the day we lost our son, my husband and I visit the cemetery. He's buried in the children's section, and since it's right after Halloween, there are always lots of decorations on the graves. There's a statue of an angel, and I think about her watching over all these tiny souls. Afterward, we go for a long walk in the forest preserve. Somehow, being in nature feels like the right thing to do. It's been ten years. I can't believe it because it seems so close. I can remember the day we lost him so clearly. I think about him all the time. Somehow, the time has passed, and we have traveled with it.

BRITTANY

Even after more than ten years, both my husband and I take our son's birthday off work. It is such a bittersweet remembrance, and we are still unsure how our emotions will be on that day. Often the most difficult days are in the week before, and then on his birthday, we can be more at peace. We try to treat ourselves gently that day. It is in the dead of winter, mid-February, so we also try to make plans for the spring and summer on that day. Looking to the future has been helpful for us. On more than one anniversary, we have gone to the ballpark and bought a few games of baseball tickets for the coming months.

Independent of where your future finds you on a birth or death date anniversary or every October, you can plan ways to reflect, whether in thought, word (journal entry or a poem), or through action (visiting the cemetery or taking a walk in nature). Through your reflections, even if they occur in your mind alone, you will ensure your prior pregnancy or deceased baby is never forgotten.

Remember

Regardless of your faith or spiritual background or upbringing, you may also explore ways to establish various traditions that hold meaning and provide comfort.

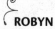
ROBYN

We are of the Jewish faith, so traditionally we honor our daughter by lighting a yahrzeit (memorial) candle on the anniversary of her death and Jewish holidays. We also did an unveiling of her headstone about a year after her funeral. Although that was another painful experience, it gave me some peace. Near her graveside, there is a giant willow tree. I think about this beautiful tree often. I believe it protects her and watches over her in a way I can never do. Most important, we honor her by living our lives to the fullest. We enjoy parenting her handsome, bright older brother, and her adorable, feisty little sister. She will always be a part of our family and in my heart forever.

JENNY

I feel like the challenging and not straight road to grow our family has given me such a greater perspective on pregnancy, humanity, and existence in general! When things don't go right, you realize how many things can go wrong, and then it seems almost impossible that it can ever go right! I have such a greater appreciation for the true miracle that is life and feel like I can love and appreciate my living babies with that deeper sense of awe and gratitude. I also have a much greater sense of empathy for others whose path is not straight. There is comfort in that camaraderie of heartbreak.

As far as remembering goes, it was meaningful at the time, and to this day, that after losing our baby during pregnancy we decided to name him. That act felt like a recognition of love and gave him a forever role in our family. We had a little ceremony to mark his existence. We invited a handful of people who were close to us and who had supported us. We planted two trees—one for him and one for his living brother—so neither one of them would ever be alone. My husband and I each wrote letters that we buried under our baby's tree during the planting, and we said some words of remembrance and love. We made copies of the letters and keep them to this day in a box with other mementos of him. We also still include his name in our nightly family prayers.

AUBREY

One thing we've done to honor our babies is to get tattoos. [My husband] has the triplets' initials and birth year, and mine is six flying birds on my arm for all six of my babies. I wanted to honor all of them—the three who are no longer living, and the three that helped bring my heart back to life.

The loss of the triplets has changed me in so many ways and continues to influence my life. I suspect that will be the case forever. I am not afraid of facing challenges and hard things. I know my own strength now, and I embrace it. I also know that life is not entirely in my control, and I have learned to accept that and anticipate it. And I see how life is short and unpredictable, and I want to live it—fully, and with as much passion, love, and emotion as I can.

Remembrances are highly individual, as evidenced by some women who create memorial gardens, wear jewelry commemorating their baby's birthstone, recognize birthdays and anniversaries, hold on to physical mementos, release butterflies, plant a tree, or simply carry their remembrances in their hearts. In time, you will find what works best for you, and again, that may vary from year to year. These are personal decisions that should be made without judgment and guilt.

Reach Out

Even if your instinct is to express your remembrances more privately, you still may consider reaching out to others and establishing a connection with the larger community around you. This may be accomplished through a financial donation that helps support research or to an organization you designate in honor or memory of your deceased baby. It may be via a note of support and love to someone you know who has experienced a loss, or it may be a message of gratitude to someone who helped you during your own time of loss. It may even be as simple as surrounding yourself with people most meaningful to you to ensure you remain supported and not alone.

MARNEY

I feel like I have become more grateful. I am aware of how fragile life can be, and I try always to let the people around me know how much I love them. I am definitely stronger. The day-to-day drama does not affect me as much, and finally, I have become much more empathic. I find myself reaching out to people (whether I know them or not) to support them after a loss. I feel like they need to know that there will eventually be a light at the end of the tunnel and that this grief will evolve and change. I want them to know that they will be able to breathe again.

Raise Awareness

Although you can bring more attention to the cause during October, your efforts don't have to be limited to that month alone. You can raise awareness about pregnancy and infant loss at any time, and in various ways, including through private/anonymous efforts (making a donation to an organization that supports children's causes), in person, and more publicly (via social media).

ERIN

Each year on our daughter's birthday, our family selects a different local nonprofit organization that benefits children. Our family makes a donation in her memory and spends part of the day visiting and volunteering with the organization.

MARY

The first year after I lost my daughter in May, I bought small lily of the valley seed packages and asked our family members and friends to plant them in memory of her. I did that because that was the flower of her birth month, and also because they are known to be associated with sweetness, motherhood, and hope.

The second year, I decided on forget-me-not flower seeds. The petals are mostly blue, but there are some varieties you can buy that have pink petals. Every year since, I do the same thing, only I share them with an increasing

number of others—even at the nursery where I buy the seeds. I package them
with a short note asking people to please plant the seeds in a new location ev-
ery year. I ask them to be planted in memory of my daughter, in honor of my
two living sons who were born after her, and now also for all other women who
have been touched by similar losses as mine. In some small way, I feel like I'm
doing my part. ⟋

Independent of the ways you find to reflect, remember, reach out, and raise
awareness now, perhaps one of the most significant and lasting remembrances
and tributes is recognizing the personal and highly positive impact you can
have as a parent to the baby in your life today. As a once-bereaved woman who
has since completed another pregnancy and birth, you embody fierce grit, per-
severance, courage, and singlehandedly illustrate all that is possible. You have
overcome darkness; you have also overcome death.

JACKIE

I think of my loss as a part of a very difficult journey, the low point but still, just
one point on a whole journey to get to where I am today with my family. I focus
on the physical child standing before me, how easy it would have been for her
not to exist, and how extraordinary her existence is. While the effects of past
traumas are mostly just shadows for me now, I know that my ability to over-
come has been tested and I survived (with the help of many amazing people!),
and that gives me great confidence. ⟋

As you continue to navigate the challenges life hands you in the years
ahead—parenting and otherwise—remember these things and practice
teaching them to your children so they may also continue to find ways to grow
and thrive through and beyond their own challenges. This is a lasting legacy
you live and will teach your children to live—all because of everything you've
experienced, and learned from your tragic, but meaningful past.

My Otherwise

(Written after the prompt of hearing "Otherwise" by Jane Kenyon)

Had the heavens not opened up
and swallowed you
it would have been
otherwise

Our path took a jarring turn over a cliff
the wheels left the rails
the way laid out before us
evaporated

Parallel realities sparred
for dominance
new roads were cut from
the vast wilderness of grief

Today your brother lights
our lives
his laughter the breath
that billows our sails

This new life
after death
no less holy than what
we would have had with you, could have had with you

Yet there are still moments
set in busy days
I wonder what would have been
Otherwise

    —BRITTANY

Acknowledgments

I must first acknowledge and thank my own children—Ellie, Celia, Alex, and Evan—to whom this book is dedicated. As deeply passionate as I am about my professional work, *you* are my life's greatest work. Each of you is an incredible and precious gift, and I am filled with gratitude for all of you daily. Every day you challenge and teach me ways to be a better mom, therapist, and person. And you fill my life with deeper love, joy, laughter, and a richness I had never known prior to your existence. You four are my absolute world.

I wish to acknowledge Dr. Nehama Dresner who is a brilliant visionary and one of the first to advocate for the role of a perinatal loss mental health professional in the hospital setting over twenty years ago, paving the way for me by helping secure funding and educating others on the need and value of this type of support. You have been a mentor for twenty years, opening many doors of opportunity—first at Northwestern Memorial Hospital, and then through invitation to join your private practice where I have continued to grow professionally. I will forever remain grateful to you for being both a mentor, and now also, a friend.

I wish to acknowledge my many interdisciplinary medical and mental health colleagues. I have learned so much from you over the years, and I treasure my relationships with all of you. I could not do the work I do without your partnerships, collaborations, and personal friendships. Thank you. Truly. On behalf of myself, and all of the patients for whom you provide care.

I wish to acknowledge my exceptional publishing team in chronological order as I met each of you. June Clark, you are an editorial, publishing, and creative consultant extraordinaire. I unexpectedly found you in New York, and now cannot imagine my life without you in it. You sincerely know every single aspect of the publishing world and impress and amaze with your keen eye, deep intellect, and unimaginable breadth of knowledge and perspective. You have provided me with ongoing honest and necessary feedback every step of the way, and also extended invaluable advice and guidance, along with resolute dedication to this project—all things that proved invaluable in helping me successfully revise my book proposal, create my website, and overhaul my original manuscript. Without your expert counsel and unwavering support, I would still be sending out queries. I'm forever grateful for our professional relationship, but so pleased to now also call you my friend. I look forward to our future collaborations together.

As to the other crucial members of my publishing team, I want to thank Stephany Evans of Ayesha Pande Literary Agency in New York, Renée Sedliar, editorial director, West Coast/Hachette Go (an imprint of Hachette Books), Alison Dalafave, Amber Morris, Iris Bass, Lauren Rosenthal, Christine Mortise, Anna Hall, and my entire team at Hachette Books. Thank you for immediately understanding and appreciating the importance of this book and being so willing to champion my messages and the women represented within. I am forever grateful to you all for your hard work, dedication, and stellar guidance through this process. I am humbled by the incredible opportunity to work with each of you and I look forward to maintaining and growing these partnerships well into the future. You are an intelligent and formidable group of professionals, for whom I have the deepest respect and admiration.

And, last, I wish to acknowledge all of my patients. You and your incredible stories have captured me and changed me. I cannot express the depth of my respect and appreciation for you, some who have generously shared parts of their stories here. I will never forget you, your families, and all of your beautiful children. I am proud of the infinitely difficult emotional work you've done to get to where you are today, and I am inspired by you all. I will always feel grateful and honored when you think to send pictures around the holidays, share images of birthday celebrations, milestone events, or just because you've captured an especially sweet moment with your child(ren). Those photos touch my heart and continue to confirm for me there is life after loss. I see it, I believe it, and I continue to celebrate it along with you. It is exactly this evidence that allows me to continue my work in this field, more passionate than ever, working to inspire and challenge others to take the leaps of faith you each did, even when they don't yet see, and certainly don't yet believe there can be rebirth. I counsel them, once, you didn't either. Thank you again to those who have shared your stories now. May they raise much-needed awareness, provide comfort, inspire hope, and encourage an ever-growing and deepening sense of peace. *You* now are the light for others.

Resources and Support

IMMEDIATE SUPPORT

National Perinatal/Postpartum Depression Hotline
1-800-PPD-MOMS (1-800-773-6667)

National Suicide Prevention Lifeline
1-800-SUICIDE (1-800-784-2433) or 1-800-273-8255 (available 24 hours every day)

PREGNANCY AND INFANT LOSS

Centering Corporation
The Centering Corporation is a nonprofit organization dedicated to providing education and resources for the bereaved—adults and children.
https://centering.org/

March of Dimes
This organization leads the fight for the health of all mothers and babies in the areas of medical research, education of pregnant women, community programs, government advocacy, and support of pregnant women and mothers.
https://marchofdimes.org/

MISS Foundation
Established in 1996, this international volunteer-based organization provides counseling, advocacy, research, and educational services (C.A.R.E) to women and their families experiencing the death of a child.
https://missfoundation.org/

National Pregnancy and Infant Loss Awareness Month

The month of October was designated by President Ronald Reagan on October 25, 1988, to recognize the loss many parents experience across the United States and around the world and to inform and provide resources for parents. Consider recognizing this month (and especially October 15) in a meaningful way to support and remember.
https://nationaltoday.com/national-pregnancy-and-infant-loss-awareness-month/

Now I Lay Me Down to Sleep

The Mission of NILMDTS is to introduce remembrance photography to parents suffering the loss of a baby with a free gift of professional portraiture, capturing love and creating a legacy.
https://www.nowilaymedowntosleep.org/

PLIDA—Pregnancy Loss and Infant Death Alliance

This organization believes that providing perinatal bereavement care is imperative. Its members serve as leaders in perinatal and neonatal bereavement care through education, advocacy, and networking for health care providers and parent advocates.
https://plida.org/

Share Pregnancy and Infant Loss Support

This is a national organization and community for anyone who has been affected by the tragic death of a baby—from parents, grandparents, siblings, and others within the family unit, to the professionals who also care for them. This organization has over seventy-five chapters in the United States and Canada, and offerings include face-to-face support groups, private online communities, memorial events, trainings for caregivers, and so on.
http://nationalshare.org/

Star Legacy Foundation

This nonprofit organization is dedicated to reducing pregnancy loss and neonatal death and improving care for the families who experience such tragedy by increasing awareness, supporting research, promoting education, and encouraging advocacy and family support.
https://starlegacyfoundation.org/

Still Standing Magazine

Founded in 2012, *Still Standing Magazine* shares stories from around the world by writers surviving the aftermath of child loss and infertility, and includes information on how others can help.
https://stillstandingmag.com/

INFERTILITY

RESOLVE

This national infertility organization supports family building by empowering individuals with knowledge, supporting them through community, uniting through advocacy, and inspiring people to act.
https://www.resolve.org

BEFORE, DURING, AND AFTER PREGNANCY

American Psychological Association: "What is postpartum depression and anxiety?"

This online printable brochure outlines the symptoms and risk factors of PPD, and provides resources and links to help.
https://www.apa.org/pi/women/resources/reports/postpartum-depression.aspx

Centers for Disease Control (CDC)

Through research, public health monitoring, scientific assistance, and partnerships, the CDC's Division of Reproductive Health (DRH) serves as the focal point for issues related to reproductive health, maternal health, and infant health, and is dedicated to improving the lives of women, their children, and their families.
https://www.cdc.gov/reproductivehealth

March of Dimes

See page 245.

MGH Center for Women's Mental Health

This center (based in Massachusetts General Hospital/Harvard Medical School) provides a range of current information including discussion of new research findings in women's mental health across the life cycle (including postpartum psychiatric disorders). This center strives to provide sound information to patients and providers alike so that individual clinical decisions can be made in a thoughtful and collaborative fashion.
https://womensmentalhealth.org/posts/is-it-postpartum-depression-or-post
partum-anxiety-whats-the-difference/

Organization of Teratology Information Specialists (OTIS)

This nonprofit organization is dedicated to providing accurate evidence-based, expert information to patients and health care professionals about exposures during pregnancy and breastfeeding.
https://mothertobaby.org

Postpartum Depression Alliance of Illinois

This site provides an excellent, consolidated online database of local programs and resources on postpartum depression throughout the state of Illinois.
https://www.ppdil.org/

Postpartum Support International

This site provides direct peer support to families, trains professionals, and provides a bridge to connect them.
http://www.postpartum.net/

US Department of Health and Human Services, Office on Women's Health: Depression During and After Pregnancy Fact Sheet

This site offers excellent basic information about the different forms of depression that may occur during a pregnancy and postpartum.
https://www.womenshealth.gov/mental-health/mental-health-conditions/post partum-depression

WOMEN'S MENTAL HEALTH

MGH Center for Women's Mental Health

See page 247.

National Institute of Mental Health

This is the lead federal agency for research on mental disorders and one that is committed to transforming the understanding and treatment of mental illness. The NIMH is part of the National Institutes of Health (NIH), the largest biomedical research agency in the world. Their mission focuses on prevention, recovery, and cure. Their website search engine is extensive and can provide more information on depression, anxiety, and post-traumatic stress, for example.
https://www.nimh.nih.gov/index.shtml

In addition to the listings provided here, many up-to-date and useful resources pertaining to infertility, pregnancy and infant loss, and women's mental health can be found on Joey Miller's website at www.joeymillermsw.com /resources.

Notes

1: FACING THE AFTERMATH OF TRAGEDY

1. https://www.statista.com/statistics/295824/us-number-of-pregnancies/.
2. https://www.cdc.gov/nchs/fastats/births.htm.
3. https://www.mayoclinic.org/diseases-conditions/pregnancy-loss-miscarriage/symptoms-causes/syc-20354298.
4. https://www.cdc.gov/ncbddd/stillbirth/facts.html.
5. https://www.cdc.gov/nchs/products/databriefs/db328.htm.
6. https://www.cdc.gov/reproductivehealth/maternalinfanthealth/pretermbirth.htm.
7. https://www.cdc.gov/reproductivehealth/maternalinfanthealth/infantmortality.htm.
8. https://www.ncbi.nlm.nih.gov/pmc/articles/PMC3909453/.
9. https://www.who.int/gho/child_health/mortality/neonatal_infant_text/en.
10. American Psychiatric Association, *Diagnostic and Statistical Manual for Mental Disorders*, 5th ed. (Washington, DC: 2013).

2: THE DEPTH AND DURATION OF GRIEF

1. Elisabeth Kübler-Ross, *On Death and Dying* (New York: Macmillan, 1969).
2. Anna Freud, *The Ego and the Mechanisms of Defense* (London: Hogarth Press and Institute of Psycho-Analysis, 1937).

3: THE WAIT (AND WEIGHT) SURROUNDING WHEN TO START TRYING

1. M. Cuisinier, H. Janssen, C. de Graauw, S. Bakker, and C. Hoogduin, "Pregnancy Following Miscarriage: Course of Grief and Some Determining Factors," *Journal of Psychosomatic Obstetrics and Gynecology* 17, no. 3 (1996), 168–174.
2. "What is recurrent pregnancy loss (RPL)?" Patient Education Website of the American Society for Reproductive Medicine (ASRM), www.reproductivefacts.org.

11: THE FIRST YEAR

1. Centers for Disease Control and Prevention, "Reproductive Health. Depression Among Women. [How many women experience depression?]," https://www.cdc.gov/reproductive health/depression/index.htm.

2. American Psychiatric Association, *Diagnostic and Statistical Manual for Mental Disorders*, 5th ed. (Washington, DC: 2013).

3. Centers for Disease Control and Prevention, "Reproductive Health. Depression Among Women. [Symptoms of postpartum depression]," https://www.cdc.gov/reproductivehealth /depression/index.htm.

4. Centers for Disease Control and Prevention, "Reproductive Health. Depression Among Women. [Risk factors for depression]," https://www.cdc.gov/reproductivehealth /depression/index.htm.

5. Rochester Mayo Clinic, "Postpartum depression. Risk factors," https://www.mayo clinic.org/diseases-conditions/postpartum-depression/basics/risk-factors/con-20029130.

6. Postpartum Support International, "Anxiety During Pregnancy & Postpartum," https://www.postpartum.net/learn-more/anxiety-during-pregnancy-postpartum.

Index

About the Author

Ms. Joey Miller, MSW, LCSW, is a licensed clinical social worker with twenty years' experience in reproductive psychology, loss and trauma, and women's mental health. She received her training and degrees from Northwestern University and Loyola University Chicago. Joey began her career working in the areas of adult trauma and emergency medicine before gaining unparalleled experience in the areas of pregnancy and infant loss while serving as the Perinatal Loss Program Coordinator at Northwestern Memorial Hospital in Chicago—the largest birthing hospital in the state of Illinois. Her work in this area is now a primary focus of her clinical practice at Wellsprings Health Associates (www.wellspringshealth.com), where she sees patients for urgent consultation and ongoing individual and couples therapy. She remains active in medical education, teaching students and training healthcare providers, and has also served as faculty at Northwestern Feinberg School of Medicine.

More information can be found on her website at
www.joeymillermsw.com.